# JUGGLiNG TWINS

## The Best Tips, Tricks, and Strategies from Pregnancy to the Toddler Years

Meghan Regan-Loomis

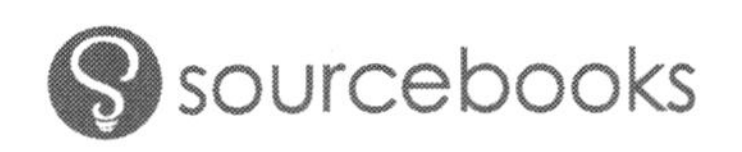

Published by Sourcebooks, Inc.
P.O. Box 4410, Naperville, Illinois 60567-4410
(630) 961-3900
Fax: (630) 961-2168
www.sourcebooks.com

Library of Congress Cataloging-in-Publication Data

Regan-Loomis, Meghan.
Juggling twins : the best tips, tricks, and strategies from pregnancy to the toddler years / by Meghan Regan-Loomis.
p. cm.
Includes index.
1. Twins—Care. 2. Twins—Psychology. 3. Infants—Care. 4. Toddlers—Care. 5. Parenting. 6. Child rearing. I. Title.
HQ777.35.R44 2008
649'.144—dc22

2008027156

Printed and bound in the United States of America.
POD 20 19 18 17 16 15 14 13 12 11 10

for Tom Loomis and Bill Regan

# Contents

# Acknowledgments

Thank you, Jen Vereker, for lending your wealth of infant twin know-how. Thank you to my students, whose hard work to improve their writing inspires me greatly. Thanks to Bill Sutherland, word-smith. Thanks, Jason and Wendy Evans, for generously sharing details of your family life, and to Paul Cremo. Our eternal gratitude to Kate Hall and her Bluebirds, who gave us precious sleep and even more precious advice. Thank you, Gail Berlinger, scrounging researcher. Thanks to my friends at the Metrowest Mothers of Twins Club. Long may you sleep. I am grateful to have had a patient, indulgent editor in Sara Appino. Thank you, my colleagues in the best high school English department in this galaxy; you inspire and dazzle me. Danielle Bartone, thank you for your tireless help with our family and for being a great friend to every one of us. Carolyn Blom, thank you for reading and for keeping me laughing. Thank you, Jennie Jacoby, my pal and my intrepid reader. Kate Sutherland, my beloved sister, thank you for reading and giving continuously, and mostly, for loving the children as we do. And thank you to my coach, my love, my RLR. I'd marry you all over again, if only we could find a free hour in which we could schedule the ceremony.

# Preface: Everywhere You Look

*Infancy conforms to nobody; all conform to it...*

—Ralph Waldo Emerson, "Self-Reliance"

When we are trying to conceive, we see pregnant women everywhere. When we are pregnant, we see babies everywhere. And when we are pregnant with twins, we see double strollers with matched sets of little ones everywhere we look. But in this case, it is not a psychological phenomenon creating the effect. You are not simply imagining that there are more twins than there used to be. In fact, the increase in multiple births over the past twenty-five years has been staggering. Since 1980, the incidence of multiple births in this country has ballooned by 70 percent. When my twins were born, they joined the ranks of 132,217 other twins born in the United States that year.[1]

So you are not alone. Not even remotely. And while that fact may for a moment seem to take the sheen off your newly minted status as a mother of twins, in no time it will become a huge comfort to you. By networking with other twin moms who have met this challenge, survived, and even thrived, you can learn the valuable lessons they have stumbled upon and taught each other as they have cared for their twin babies. This book catalogues those hard-won lessons and hopes to serve as your first mentor and coach as you embark on this challenge.

---

1. J.A. Martin, B.E. Hamilton, P.D. Sutton, S.J. Ventura, F. Menacker, S. Kirmeyer, and M.L. Munson, "Births: Final Data for 2005," *National Vital Statistics Reports* 56, no. 6 (Hyattsville, MD: National Center for Health Statistics, 2007); J.A. Martin, B.E. Hamilton, P.D. Sutton, S.J. Ventura, F. Menacker, S. Kirmeyer, and M.L. Munson, "Births: Final Data for 2004," *National Vital Statistics Reports* 55, no. 1 (Hyattsville, MD: National Center for Health Statistics, 2007).

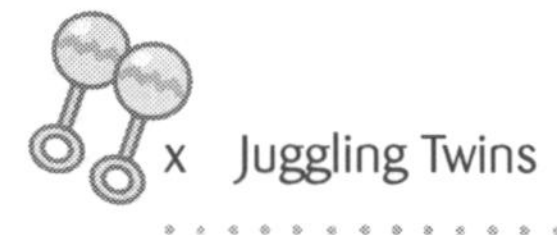


Raising twins will present trials above and beyond the already daunting tasks of "normal" parenthood, and these challenges will begin shortly after conception. Not only must you familiarize (or re-familiarize) yourself with the basics of infant care, but you also must learn the unique demands of a multiple pregnancy, birth, and infancy. The principal goal of this book is to prepare you for the latter of these. After an overview of the best current thinking on carrying and delivering twins, subsequent chapters will answer questions that are less commonly addressed directly but that can feel just as pressing for soon-to-be parents of twins: namely, *How in the world are we going to do this? How will we manage? How will it work? How will we help their sibling through this? Where will the babies sleep? When? How do we feed them? What if they're not well? When should family visit? How do we get both kids loaded into the car? Can we get them on the same schedule? Will we ever leave the house? What happens when all the help is gone?*

The intent of this book is to help you prepare for and manage the first year of having twins, as those months can be most overwhelming, exhausting, and frustrating. It is not uncommon to hear parents of twins refer to those early months as a time of crisis or triage. Beleaguered parents invoke war imagery, as "troops" of supporter-soldiers prepare for the "battle" of caring for infant twins. But good planning and the determination to approach this not as a predicament but as a challenge that calls for an active sense of humor and an upbeat attitude can make these intense months some of the most exhilarating of your life, without the need to think of them in terms of full-blown combat. This book will coach you to experience your children's infancy as a manageable campaign, offering very specific advice that, when heeded, can bring order to the chaos and allow you to focus on the blissful elements of having twins—your amazing good fortune to have been twice blessed. By approaching this chapter of your life feeling prepared and supported,

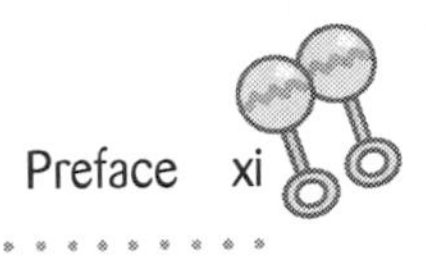

you will be able to see the management of your babies' needs not as a draining, soul-sapping proposition, but instead as a wonderful, intense challenge that draws on the best of you, creates an amplified closeness between you and your partner, and most importantly, gives your precious babies a safe and healthy start in a calm, happy, and loving home.

The stresses associated with caring for two babies are many, but they are predictable. Preparing for them with proven techniques can mean the difference between feeling relentlessly assaulted by your babies' needs and feeling the profound satisfaction of anticipating and meeting those needs. This book will help you to prepare, cope, and laugh. It is a step-by-step guide that will help you create the time and the calm to enjoy these months of your twins' infancy for what they are: a glorious gift to be treasured, not simply endured.

# Part I
# Pregnancy: On Your Mark, Get Set

Have you ever been so tired in your whole life? Just think about what you're doing every day! You are growing *two people.* Two hearts, two brains, forty digits, four eyes and ears, several hundred bones...A twin pregnancy is exceptionally challenging work on all fronts, and each trimester has its special trials. The exhaustion caused by forming multiples in the early months of pregnancy soon enough gives way to the exhaustion caused by lugging an exaggerated edition of yourself around town. And while the second trimester is easi*er* than the other two, no element can accurately be called easy.

Regardless of whether the news of your doubled expectancy was the most exhilarating or the most horrifying news you had ever received, you have no doubt been experiencing some level of anxiety in addition to the physical stresses of this pregnancy. Not only is your pregnancy more complicated than most, by definition, but you also just might be worried about how you will handle the next... well, the next twenty or so years to follow.

Relax. All will be well. By focusing on small chunks at a time—days and weeks, rather than months and years—you will be able from the start to exert some control over your life even as the impending arrival of two babies threatens to turn everything you know completely upside down and inside out. Step by step, you can bring quite a lot of order to a situation that, left on its own, embodies chaos in its purest form. Those deliberate steps can begin now, and the sooner, the better. While you are gestating these babies, you can also be gestating some plans. Some of them can come to fruition even before the babies do.

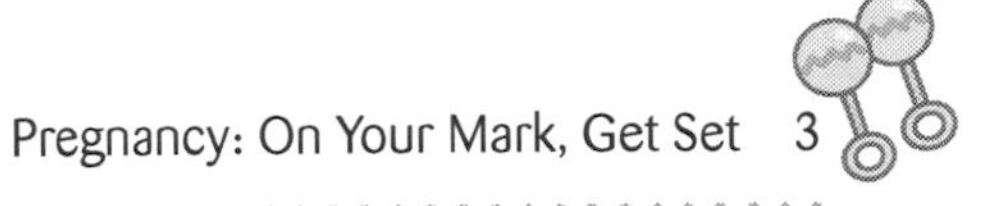

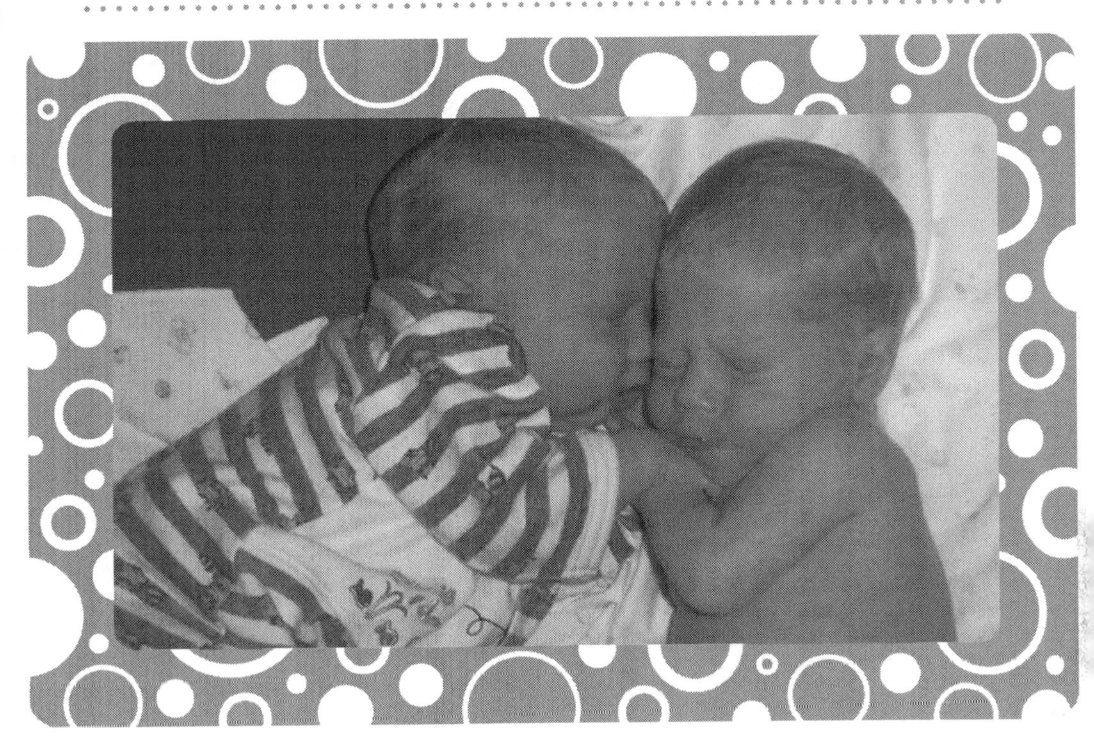

Ready or not, here they come…

Photo courtesy of the Gearys

# 1

# Getting Them Close to Term

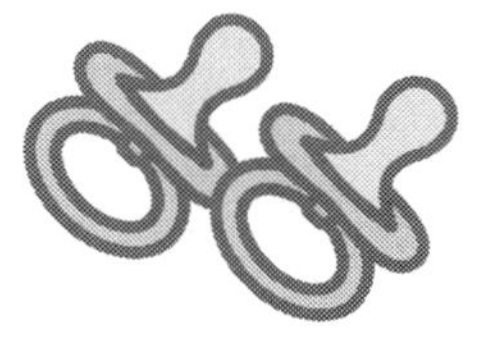

In my twin travels since having our boys, I have met so many families with multiples who have moving, sometimes tragic, sometimes nearly heroic stories about childbirth: the setting is usually the NICU, and the protagonists, two or three tiny babies who come much too early. Neonatal care has become astoundingly effective, and many of these stories now end happily after a frightening start and much arduous effort. But even when all seems well after the crisis period of weeks or months in the hospital, the lingering tragedy of the hidden harm produced by an early birth remains, and the eventual emergence of these problems is a slow drip of agonized worry and coping over years, whether the problems are as mild as slight learning differences or as severe as cerebral palsy.

It is a difficult project for a woman's body, be it twenty-four years old or forty-three years old, to grow more than one baby at once and take them to term. Actually, it's a pretty tall order to do so with *one* baby. As common as having multiples is becoming, it is tempting for us to think that because everyone seems to be doing it, it must be a reasonable proposition. But in spite of the numbers of us having twins or more, it remains a daunting task right from the first trimester. While it obviously can be done, it is worthwhile to bear in mind that we weren't truly designed to make two at a time. We cannot simply assume that our bodies will figure out what needs to be done and obligingly provide, regardless of the level of our more conscious efforts.

Dr. Barbara Luke's book, *When You're Expecting Twins, Triplets, or Quads* (coauthored with Tamara Eberlein, published by Harper Collins, 1999), is a great resource for helping to ensure a healthy multiple pregnancy and delivery. When I was pregnant, we read it, re-read it, highlighted it, re-re-read, and marked important passages with stickies. It was completely dog-eared by the end of my pregnancy. In a nutshell, the author, who is a prominent researcher in prenatal nutritional issues, argues for the importance of substantial maternal weight gain in order to bring multiples to term. But please don't be contented with the nutshell version. Go get the book.

## Eat More and Slow Down

The truth is that you can do a lot to increase your chances of getting your babies to term. Ironically, the most important elements to success are two ideas that have become completely counterintuitive for the modern western woman: to eat more and to slow down. Very quickly, you need to reorient your thinking so that you can see weight gain and rest as *good things,* even if they have been your tacit enemies since adolescence. The concept of needing more rest when gestating two babies would seem self-evident at some level, and yet most of us are so accustomed to catapulting ourselves through hectic, overscheduled days and into evenings of re-grouping, bill paying, housecleaning, and scheduling tomorrow's madness that "rest" or "slowing down" means doing all that except, perhaps, the dishes. It's difficult for us to imagine how life would proceed if we truly eliminated or lessened the activities that fill our days. The dry cleaning can't get itself. That disgusting bathtub won't self-clean. One ought to pay one's bills. Right? Sort of.

Yes, life goes on. But your contributions to operations of the household must, must, must be diminished, and this is true even if you love being pregnant and have never felt better in your life. This is not simply a remedy for the suffering. It is a preemptive measure

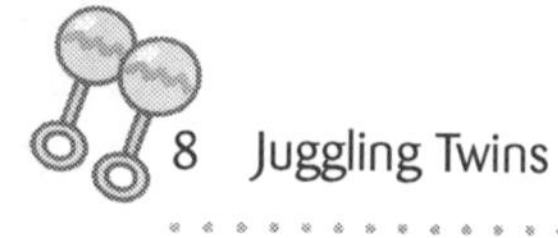


that will help ensure the babies' health. You need to rest every day, and at times of the day that would normally embarrass you as indulgences. This means a nap after lunch, or as soon as you get home from work, and an early—as in right after dinner—bedtime, even if you lie in bed and read for hours before sleeping. Even if you feel capable of pushing harder and getting more done, don't. If you wait until you are totally beat and aching to rest, you have waited too long. It's like getting an oil change for the car: if you can feel a difference in your drive afterward, you waited too long. This is preventative rest, not restorative rest. And someone else will simply have to pick up the slack on everything else from bathtub scrubbing to board meetings. You will probably be surprised to see how much

## Reality Check

Research points repeatedly to rest and nutrition as crucial in determining the health of twin babies. Yet as convinced as I was by the logic of this research, I still struggled with the notion of pursuing a substantial weight gain. That is, at the same time that I was willingly and healthfully gaining seventy pounds over thirty-nine weeks, I was simultaneously sickened by the thought that perhaps I would only lose, say, eleven pounds of it. I had a hard time believing faithfully in my being able to lose that much, having struggled with my weight in the past. This was a strange emotional position to occupy: half of my brain saying, "Eat. *Eat!*" and the other half saying, "Oh Lord, will I weigh over two hundred pounds for the rest of my life?" The answer for me was no; in fact, I weigh less now than I have since high school. (My high school friends will tell you that this isn't terribly impressive, which is just one of the many reasons I no longer hang out with them...but you see my point, right?) Gaining more weight than your entire body weighed in fourth grade needs to become a goal, not a dread.

more adaptable others are to your new status as a slug, compared to you yourself. Give yourself permission to give these babies the best chance they can have, knowing that it involves some sacrifices.

Eat as much healthful, protein-filled, vitamin-packed food as you can manage. And then eat more. And then take a nap. There are all sorts of reasons that multiples sometimes come early, so it is simply incorrect and unfair to surmise that a mother of preemies didn't do everything she could to get those babies to term. At the same time, eating and sleeping are two behaviors that you *can* control that will help to give your babies the best possible chance they have to stay where they belong until they are fully cooked. As we used to say during my third trimester: in spite of the aching back and sleep disturbances, they are much, much easier to take care of while they're still inside you.

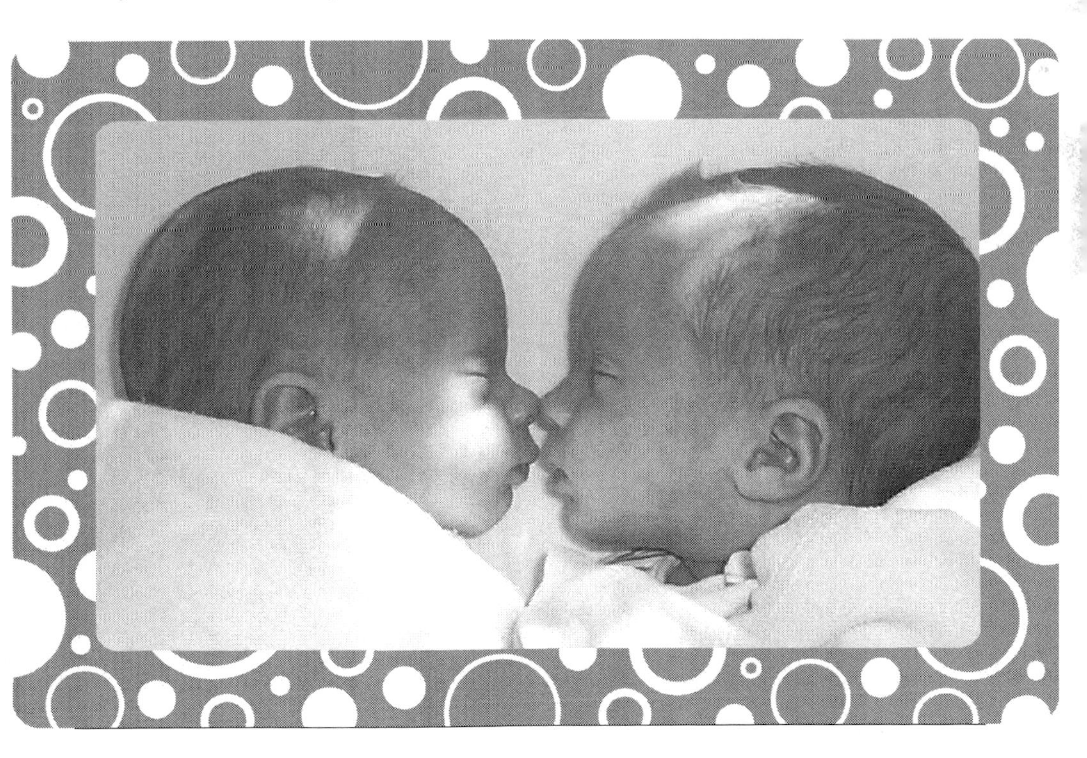

Two-week old, full-term twins

Photo courtesy of Roger and Marielle Horstmann

# 2

# The Diaper Party

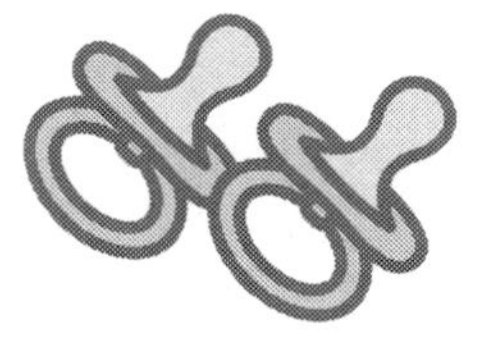

Of all the advice you will receive in this book, this may be the one piece that you will be most grateful for having heeded, and your gratitude will emanate straight from your wallet. It is advice that will be easier to follow if you have already had a child, but please try to have faith in it even if these are your first babies.

Although twins are increasingly common, they are still special. In fact, they routinely produce in bystanders a sort of awe-filled intrigue. Given that this is the case with strangers, imagine the captivation of those you know and love. Your family and friends will be fascinated and charmed by the idea of your twins from the day you announce that you are expecting them, and that focused affection will be even more intense if your twins are the happy answer to months or years of infertility struggles. Your village can't help but dance with delight. And the bearing of gifts will be a primary expression of this elation. Whether these are your first and second children or your ninth and tenth (makes you cringe just to read that, doesn't it?), you will be inundated with gifts for them, in part because there is such novelty to their multiplicity.

Stop it right in its tracks.

Before the gifts start rolling in, explain that you aren't accepting traditional gifts, because there is a plan in the works that will require the gift-bearers' financial participation elsewhere. If you are too embarrassed or tasteful to throw yourself a party, then you need to enlist the help of a friend to act as if this were entirely his or her idea. Go to the person who was most likely to throw you a shower. And here's what you do: instead of a traditional shower, you're going to have a cocktail party. Or a barbecue. Or an elaborate dinner party, or a bowling party, or a pub crawl. Whatever sort of grown-up party you most enjoy. And it will be big. This needs in fact to be the biggest party you've ever thrown, with invitations going out to everyone you've ever liked even remotely until you have sent out enough to fill your house twice with guests. The catch is that nobody gets in the door without a case of diapers.

## Diaper Economics

Here's the reasoning. On average, a single diaper costs more than twenty-five cents, even when bought in bulk. Babies go through anywhere from six to twelve diapers a day. Each. So let's figure on average that you will go through eighteen or so diapers a day at more than a quarter each. That's over $1,600 a year in diapers alone for at least three years. (If that makes your knees buckle, wait until you see the formula for formula!) Obviously, diapers are not an optional purchase. Whereas you don't *need* matching sailor suits that get worn once or a third quilted floral diaper bag, you really do *need* diapers. Yes, you will need some baby equipment and some little clothes. But, for reasons that will be explored in the next chapter, you don't need to squander all your gift chits on these things. They are better spent on something for which you absolutely will otherwise be spending money. Lots of it.

In spite of all that the diaper companies do to convince us that babies pee differently according to gender and time of day and that diapers that turn colors can potty train your kid, the fact is that except for the extremely cheap sorts, diapers are pretty much diapers, and they pretty much do the same thing they always have. Also, diapers keep. They don't have an expiration date (as formula does...so don't be tempted to have a formula party, you clever one-upper, you). The size 6 diapers your tennis partner brings to the

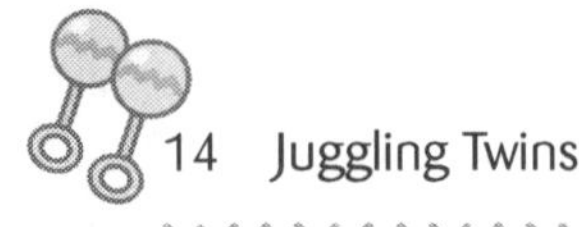



party will work perfectly fine on your three-year-olds after sitting in the attic for thirty-six months.

So you have this party. If you are like us, you make it a grown-up party with great food and music, plentiful drinks, and very few pastels, baby-bottle balloons, or teddy bear cakes. This abstention from the traditionally sentimental baby shower, besides being more fun, has a corollary benefit of involving far more men—and not only will that make for a more inclusive, enjoyable time, but you also will find that some of them are truly grateful to be involved in such a palatable manner. There needn't be one "oooh" or "ahhh," nor will anyone be subjected to watching you open seventy gifts consecutively. And the next morning, you will have in your home a stack of diaper cases with which you could build a fortress. When we did this, we amassed 5,180 diapers and 3,220 wipes. As a result, *we didn't have to buy one single diaper for nearly two years.* This plan obviously has a huge and shameless economic benefit. Less obvious now, but perhaps as beneficial down the road, is the convenience of being able to go up to the attic every time one needs a case of diapers rather than out to the nearest Costco. The idea is not simply that you will want to cut down on errands in the next couple of years because you'll be overextended; it's also that a case of diapers is not an easily carried item when pushing a twin stroller and it certainly doesn't fit in the little basket underneath.

Now, here's the über-secret to this secret plan, and God help me if any of our friends ever read this: you'll get those other gifts, anyway!

You'll have all the baby monitors, OshKosh overalls, and little leather booties you could ever use. Refer please to the previously mentioned general exuberance over twins. Your party will be, say, at the beginning of month seven or so, when you're showing impressively but still probably able to make the party and stay awake through it like a big girl (and you will be a big, big girl). Then in eight to twelve weeks, news will filter to these dear partygoers that the babies have arrived. Do you really think they're going to be contented having simply given you a stupid case of diapers? No, no, no! They will be pulled zombielike by unknown forces to their nearest Baby Gap to buy you coordinating onesies with teddy bears on the bums. Rest assured, you will not be left alone with naked babies and a huge wall of diapers.

## Party Logistics

In the invitation to the party, be sure to specify that it is in lieu of a shower (if someone gives you one anyway, well, what's a girl to do?). Explain your reasoning: the relentlessness of the need for diapers and the fact that you want to have a party at which both men and women can have a genuinely good time celebrating the impending births. Ask guests to express their gift-giving creativity through their choice of *size,* rather than *their choice of gift,* explaining that eventually you will need everything from "newborn" to size 6. One clever guest whom we had never even met before our party (as I said, throw that net out wide!) brought a "poo poo platter" loaded with diapering accessories. Let guests choose their favorite brand. You can't afford to be picky, and having tried them all on my kids, I can tell you that they are all really effective, assuming you have the kid in the right size and you know how to put the thing on correctly.

At the party, be sure to pile the cases in some very conspicuous place, like on the front porch or in the middle of the living room, so that folks can watch the pyramid grow. It will be an easy icebreaker for people who don't otherwise know one another, and since you have invited everyone from your postal delivery person to your boss's ex-husband's dermatologist, there may be few people who actually do know one another. Sick as we are, the "party game" we most enjoyed at our Diaper Party was the "Should We Circumcise?" Straw Poll and Comment-Writing Area, which was essentially a huge piece of poster board with the question at the top and a Sharpie pen tied to the side. The activity had an interesting, incendiary effect on conversations between our friends who were meeting for the first time. At the beginning of the evening, we found our co-workers engaged in serious conversations with our neighbors over the aesthetic and social aspects of this thorny issue. By the end of the evening, with the flow of alcohol slowing to a moderate ooze, men were describing their most private selves and women, their most private preferences. Let me emphasize that you are welcome to take a more mature approach to this entire party. Feel free to make it an elaborate church choir practice or a Tupperware party with a twist. In fact, you could make it a traditional shower but request only diapers. The only essential is the no diapers/no admittance rule.

An e-mail to the whole crowd the next morning with a picture of the final haul and a total count on individual diapers will be another reminder of the fun and, if you're truly efficient, will serve nicely as a group thank you. On our boys' first birthday, we sent the picture of the stacks out again but also attached another picture, this one of our big boys standing next to the remaining cases, laughing. At that point, there were still about a dozen cases left, all in appropriate sizes. We, too, were still chuckling at our own brilliance.

# 3

# Begging, Borrowing, and Stealing

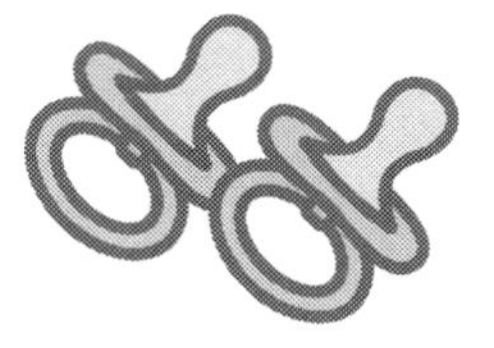

An Internet joke was forwarded to me a few years ago with one of those titles like "FW: FW: FW: FW: FW: FW: FW: FW: FW: This made me LOL—for moms." It was a simple formula that said, "First baby, her precious, just-washed clothes get changed if she appears to drool. Second baby wears hand-me-down clothes that get changed if there is verifiable spit up. Third kid—boys can wear pink, right? Fourth child, as long as it's May–October, a diaper will do; clothes just slow the diaper-changing process..." etc. I didn't LOL so much as nod; these are simple truths.

For most mothers, regardless of the current age of their children, there is something powerfully intoxicating, addictive, and symbolic about baby clothing. Before motherhood, fantasies about having children often involve dressing them in tiny clothes. The choosing of the coming-home-from-the-hospital outfit is nearly a rite of passage. Organizing the clothes that have already appeared as gifts before the birth, washing them in sweet-smelling baby detergent, folding them lovingly into the drawers of a pastel-colored dresser—all are parts of a mysteriously powerful ritual that begins during pregnancy but retains its resonance for years afterward.

One gets attached with a hormone-fueled tenderness to the clothes of the firstborn baby or babies. A mother remembers not only by whom particular pieces were given, but also what the baby wore on specific outings and the feel of individual outfits. Some mothers even save squares of their babies' outfits to fashion into quilts that can be clutched while waiting for "baby" to arrive home from prom sixteen years later. Surely there is a magnetic symbolism in the very smallness of the clothes both at the beginning, for the pregnant woman trying to imagine the clothes filled with her child, and later, for the mother of a grown child trying to imagine how he or she was ever tiny enough to fit into them.

It is therefore ridiculous to instruct a first-time parent who is having twins that she should keep the tags on all these cherished items so that she can take them all right back to the store and trade them in for diapers. Far be it for me to fight the hormonal tide. However, I will suggest that you at least refrain from removing any tags until you are actually ready to use a piece of clothing. In spite of your having told everybody, "Really, we just want diapers," there will be clothing gifts, in part because a mother's love for baby clothes applies not just to those of her own children. Shopping for baby clothes can be a spiritual experience for women at any point in their lives, and your pregnancy has doubled the potential nirvana of the women in your life. They will need to shop. So my advice is this: because most people will give you size 0–3 month clothes or, at best, size 3–6 month clothes, and because that is when you will least need them, you will probably end up taking some back, re-gifting them, trading them up for a bigger size, or saving them for your next child. So keep those tags on until that last possible moment (remembering of course that you ought to wash them before putting them next to that amazingly perfect baby skin).

## Hand-Me-Downs?

If you already have a child or children, the situation is slightly different. In the first place, you will probably receive fewer gifts, as

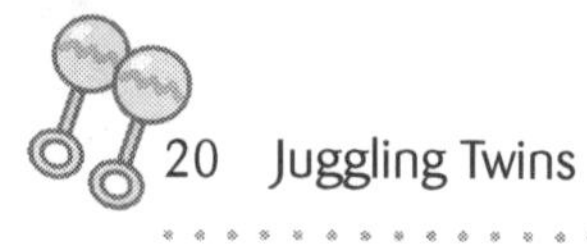


second babies and beyond typically do. But additionally, because of the twin factor, you will likely acquire bounteous hand-me-downs and hand-me-overs. If your days as a thirty-something are fading or finished, as is common for many moms of twins and for me as well, you will find that friends who have wrapped up their baby-making will see you as a worthy recipient of 95 percent of the contents of their just-cleaned attics and nurseries. Take every bit of it with a big, gratitude-soaked smile. Hopefully, they will dump the stuff on you in some sort of order, but don't count on it. Get yourself ten or twelve big plastic bins and label them with specific ages and seasons. Get them in order in your attic or basement, and as the minivans unload onto your front porch, you will be able simply to toss clothes into their appropriate bins so that when your babies grow out of a size, you need only pull down the next bin to see what your kids will be wearing that season.

Some parents just have a hard time putting their kids in used clothes. Although I'm not one of them, I do understand this at some level. I think, though, that it's an inclination worth fighting. Baby clothes, in particular, deserve recycling. Other than occasional staining and that weird tendency of seemingly clean clothes to turn yellow when stored, most baby clothes can go through many, many children before showing any wear because, let's face it, little babies *don't do much.* How can a four-month-old wear out a romper? Four-month-olds don't romp. In later years, knees blow out and elastic loses its *boing,* and issues of style may even come into play as your five-year-old points out that, *really, Mom, none of the other kids are wearing knickers to kindergarten.* But baby clothes are an easy hand-me-down, if you can get over yourself and your feeling that your prince and/or princess must have only the best. As with much of the advice in this book, this is about the long-term pacing of funds. They say the ability to delay gratification is a mark of maturity. Show your babies what a grown-up you are by delaying your gratification until eighteen years from now, when your practicality has over the years fattened that college fund. Again, this is a much easier proposition to swallow for the repeat-performance parent. New parents may only be able to get as far as leaving the tags on for a while.

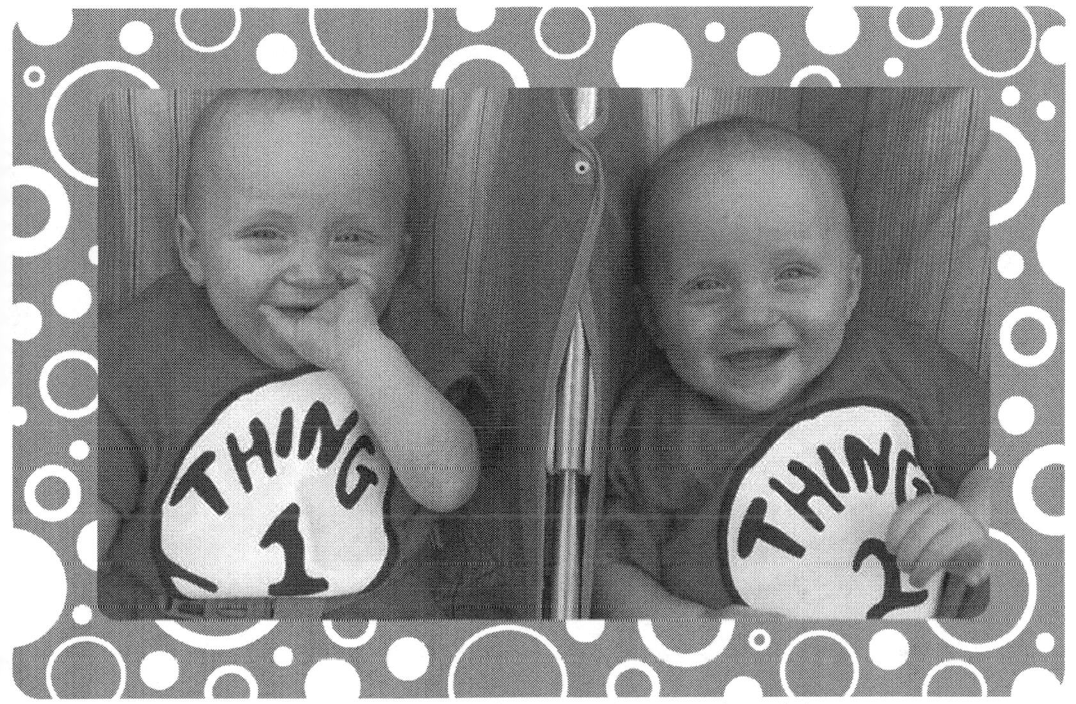


Even if you simply must dress your twins in matching clothes, you can still get creative at differentiating them.

Photo courtesy of the Regan-Loomis family

It may be easier—*may be*—for new parents to follow this wait-and-see attitude about equipment, since bouncy seats and bottle warmers can't really carry the emotional weight of a baptismal gown from Aunt Helen. In any case, the advice holds true in this arena as well. There is no need to open a brand new Diaper Champ if your neighbor is offering you the one she was going to take to the dump. They all get smelly eventually; the unsoiled new one that your book club buys you will be marked with the acrid smell of baby pee in no time. So spray your neighbor's with disinfectant, take the new one back, and

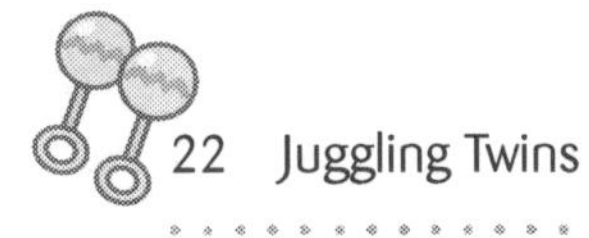


get on with it. The cloth parts of bouncy seats and exersaucers pop out and wash easily. High-end strollers should go through several rounds of kids before being trashed and can be bought secondhand if you don't know someone who is finished with a double stroller. And for later, you know that molded plastic stuff that clutters the suburban American backyard landscape? You should be ashamed if you drop a dime on it anywhere but at a yard sale. Buy the power-washer to clean it up, but don't buy the plastic playhouse.

The only pieces of equipment that you probably want to make sure you get new or in tip-top shape are the car seats. Not only does the technology improve over time (the LATCH system was devised between the births of our kids, for example), but also, the plastic molding on the snap-in mechanisms can wear out with use, so you do want to have new car seats. This is an item you should let the big spenders in your crowd—either your parents or a group of friends—go for, if they are so inclined. It is also nice to have new bottles, but new nipples are all you really need if you have bottles from friends or from an older child. Of all the equipment you will need, car seats and bottles are the only items you might not want to inherit from friends or family, but you can, if you are careful to see that they are in good shape.

# 4

# Gathering the Troops (Your Helpers)

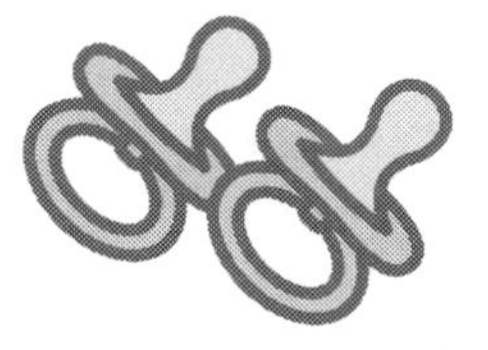

Everyone who has ever witnessed, written about, produced, or cared for twins advises parents who are expecting a pair to "get some help." Most go on to insist that you need to swallow your pride and realize that you simply can't do it alone... at least not for long. Hear, hear. It's all true. But what does that *mean?* What *sort* of help? To help with *what* exactly? Are we talking about volunteers? Paid help? Live in? Live out? For the twins or for you? To take your four-year-old to swim lessons or to change size 1 diapers? And with what money, by the way? And what if you're going to be breastfeeding? There's not a lot anyone can do to help you there unless wet nurses come back into style, right?

Before one even discusses the complex organizational grid of assignments, expectations, and scheduling, we need to consider the volume of labor to be accomplished in the first eight to twelve weeks. Seasoned parents will habitually say to novices, "You can't really be prepared," and a whole host of other condescending, vaguely terrifying truisms. As with all truisms, they are true. However, it is also true that you will find a way to muddle through, just as other parents have on their way to becoming high and mighty and so dramatically put-upon.

## Give Yourself a Break

Let's first put this in some perspective. If we were to amass a list of the Things That Need to Happen in a Household with Twins in Order to Keep Things Running Smoothly, you might despair. But don't. Think of it this way: if you were to create a list of the things that need to happen in your household every day *now* in order for you to be able to sleep at night with a sense that your life is not in total turmoil, you would probably be astounded by how much you already do routinely. The list would include not just whatever work it is that brings income to the home, but also the supplying of the home, the paying of the bills to supply it, the cleaning of it, the maintenance of the outside areas that keep growing or getting snowed upon, the physical upkeep and personal grooming of the inhabitants, the repair of vehicles, and the endless Sisyphean cycle of cooking and cleaning up after meals. What tends to surprise parents of newborns isn't so much their level of neediness or even the persistence of that need. No, what stymies new parents is their newborns' utter lack of regard for the fact that *they were already really busy* and are now adding child care to a list that already felt like plenty to do.

So in addition to all the elements of your life that normally make you fall into bed exhausted, you are now adding the obviously intense needs of two infants. It is difficult to overstate the relentlessness of the babies' needs as newborns or to explain how unconcerned infants are with fairness when it comes to the timing, duration, or occasional inexplicability of their needs. In addition to this relentlessness is the fact that the household not only ought to be maintained but also that if it is, you and the babies will have a much more peaceful and pleasant world in which to adjust to your life together.

For the most part, babies seem truly confused as to how or why they must suddenly live outside of the womb, having had it so good on the inside. As they acclimate to life on the outside, they live in a disconcerted, chaotic state. Having your world ordered will help you to order theirs. It is the combination of dealing with both—your world and theirs—that compels people to advise you to get help, because even if you were in possession of the amount of energy needed to perform every task on a daily basis (you're not, and by the way, you never will be), there isn't enough time in the day to do so. Simple logistics point to the impossibility of handling everything yourself or even handling everything as a twosome. You'll need some help at the beginning.

## Free Help: Family and Friends

Before you determine what help you may need to hire, figure out how much free help you can scrounge up. If you have capable parents, a mother-in-law, or a sister or aunt type available to help, you need to ask these people directly and clearly for commitments to being with you during parts of the first months. Get pledges of dates and times. Similarly, when friends proclaim that they will help, your answer can't be, "That's great! Thanks!" It needs to be, "When?" or better still, "Good. I need you the afternoon of the 12th from 1 p.m. to 5:30. See you then. Bring dinner." Once you are into your third trimester, have a calendar that is dedicated to nothing but the assignment of helpers. Get commitments from people who plan to visit, whether for a half hour or half a month. Any time that people can give you during the first three months is valuable. But it needs to be scheduled.

It makes a lot of sense to invite someone who knows her way around a baby to visit during those first weeks, so that the caring of the babies can be shared by you, your partner, and someone who can relieve you for a feeding, hold a sleeping baby, or if she is interested in applying for sainthood, take an overnight shift. At the same time, if your baby-shy brother wants to come help, that can work, too, as long as he is willing to do some laundry, run errands, or mow the lawn. Every day. It is not crucial that your visitors have any skill with or even interest in babies, as long as they are capable of doing some of the tasks associated with the household and its upkeep. If your parents or in-laws are able to help you, the early weeks are a great time for them to visit, but *not all at the same time,* not even if they have all been great pals since doing the macarena together at your wedding reception.

Spread the wealth of help. Have people come no more than two at a time. If they themselves are high-maintenance, they are absolutely ineligible for first-month visits. You cannot be thinking about how your mother-in-law needs clean sheets on her bed and another bottle of vermouth when what you really need is to have her run to the store to buy you bigger maxi pads. The more days on that three-month calendar that you can fill with overnight family visitors, local friends who can promise a few hours on a given date, or volunteer church or synagogue members who can commit to once a week, the fewer the blank dates for which you will need to hire someone to come in. Again, the twofold goal is to have some sort of help every day in the beginning so that, by about month three, you can handle the whole show on your own.

While the help of loved ones is a beautiful thing, it is perhaps less reliable than the kindness of strangers—that is, strangers whom you pay. Once you have scheduled all the free help and out-of-town labor, it's time to figure out when you still need some coverage. There is a myriad of possibilities as to how to proceed at this point, depending on budget, preferences, the existence of other children, and your plans for feeding the babies. (That means *how* you will feed them, not *whether* you will.) Assuming for the moment that your partner will be taking at least a week or two off from work after the births, the first priority is to be certain that someone is scheduled to help at least once every twenty-four-hour period after that during the first weeks that you are otherwise alone with the babies. It is ideal to have three adults on hand at the very beginning: you, your partner, and that third set of hands, whoever's they may be. Once the vacation time dries up, it will be down to you and a helper. That is manageable for the next couple of months, as long as those helpers keep showing up at some point in every twenty-four-hour period.

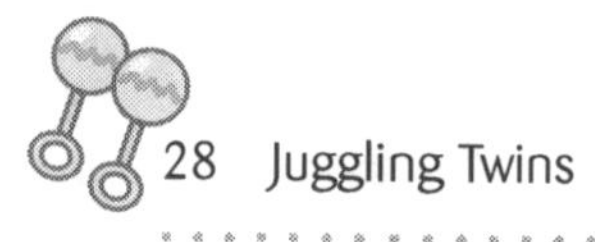


## Hired Help: Do It if You Can

Not everyone is comfortable with the idea of hired help. It may be an easier concept to swallow if you have been used to the bustling, parallel presence of cleaners in your home since you were yourself a toddler than if you have never hired someone to do anything in your home that didn't require a permit or a license. You may struggle in general with the notion of paying anyone to serve you in any capacity, or you may simply be uncomfortable with the notion of sharing such an intimate time of your life with a stranger whom you are paying. Perhaps you dread sharing your space or sacrificing the privacy you require when wearing holey pajamas or looking tousled. Or you may be all for it but simply wondering how in the world you can possibly come up with the money that this sort of help might require. You and your partner may or may not be on the same page about whether help is needed or deserved, or how much you can afford. In all, it's a concept that's never as simple as people make it sound when they advise you to "get some help."

The best advice I have for getting over your bourgeois guilt and your financial fears is to remind yourself that these are exceptional and short-lived circumstances. The critical time for lining up help is during the first three months. If by that point you have run out of either the stomach or the money for continued help, you will probably be able by then to manage on your own, particularly if you set that benchmark as a goal, as in: by three months, I want to be able to do this without any help or (many) anti-depressants. It's a reasonable goal, and one that having ample help at the beginning can actually help you meet.

Meanwhile, however, this will be very expensive. Prepare for the cost as best you can, as early as you can, understanding that as outrageous an assault on your budget as it may seem, it is *not a luxury* any more than expensive medical care or car repairs are luxuries. Even if your partner is totally on board and can be home to help care for the twins, it is *still* essential that you have help, and the scenario of a completely available partner who doesn't have to tend to a job is rare. If you are accustomed to living frugally, the rates you will need to pay good help will make you gasp and fall into reveries about how you made 25 cents an hour babysitting for Mrs. Sweeney's children. We are not talking about babysitting, though. We are talking about a professional who is better at handling these babies than you are. You can expect to pay over $100 per day or over $200 per night for this service. (I heard that. I told you you'd gasp.) Find a way. Ask your parents. Get a second mortgage. Become an escort for freaks with Madonna fetishes. Anything. But you need to convince yourself and your partner that it's not a question of whether or not you hire help. It's just a question of who and when.

Pretending for a moment that you have unlimited funds, your ideal arrangement of hired help would include a full-time nanny during the day as well as an overnight nanny. As that's not even a remote possibility for most of us, you'll need to make a decision about the type of help you hire. If you do have unlimited funds, the whole discussion of budgeting baby help becomes moot, and you should skip this section entirely and hire round-the-clock help. As for the rest of us, the idea is to look at the money available, once you have ransacked every piggy bank and rainy-day fund in the household, and then parse the funds out as evenly as possible over the first three months of the babies' lives.

## Days or Nights?

The first major decision about hired help becomes whether to hire someone for the days or the nights. Some moms of twins have suggested that one's dollar goes further with day help, which is about half the rate of overnight help, and that it therefore makes more sense to hire help for daytime and handle the nights without any employees roaming the halls. This does make some economic sense, particularly if you are a napper who could make up for lost sleep during the day with a nanny present.

The perfect day nanny would be someone who does not object to doing some housework and who is equally comfortable with infants and any older children you have. She would also be a decent cook who could willingly throw a meal together when you are nursing at the dinner hour and doesn't pucker her lips in distaste if also asked to clean up the kitchen afterwards. While these women are out there, the challenge is finding one and being able to afford her services. Your efforts to find a nanny within your budget who can take care of both the household and the children will be worth it.

Of course, it also wouldn't hurt if your nanny were super fun and unattractive, so that your toddler falls for her but your mate does not; at least thirty years old and over the bar scene, so that she doesn't show up late or hung over; in possession of enough English to know what "poopy" and "spit up" are; and willing to be coach of the team when your ass is dragging, but varsity captain when you're in good shape and again ready to bark orders. Hey, a girl can dream.

Be thoughtful about how you go about finding and hiring this help. During the day, flexibility is key. While it makes perfect sense to hire a baby expert for night shifts, for example, hiring someone for the day who will only deal with the babies and won't have anything to do with the occasional lunch dishes could mean that you end up paying someone to rock your babies while you scrub pots. This exchange of jobs could be exactly what you want and need, but there's a pretty good chance it's not. Ideally, your helper could take on all manner of assignments: handle both babies while you play with your toddler or take her to a playground; care for one baby while you run an errand with the other; do laundry while you and the babies nap; or help you throw together a meal, each of you with a baby strapped to you. Similarly, if you have another child or more, hiring a professional *baby* nurse may limit her usefulness, as she may balk at the idea of playing Candyland with your four-year-old while you and the babies sleep.

The more willing she is to adjust, the better. But two caveats: (1) Don't expect her to do what you can't do. If you go to the mall having left her with three kids and a menu you'd like her to prepare for dinner, you should expect to see your toddler in front of the TV when you get back. (2) Don't repeatedly foist your toddler on a caretaker, no matter how good she is with toddlers or how much your child likes her. Your older child or children, no matter how well-adjusted, will need you even more than they did before these babies came to town.

At the same time that you are looking for a utility player who can perform various tasks, a certain level of experience and expertise with babies is crucial. While it's not necessary that your helper has worked with multiples before, she needs to have worked with newborns enough to be able to anticipate their needs and know the basics of keeping them comfortable. Your personality and situation come into play here, too. Are you a confident mother with a plan and a closely held philosophy concerning the handling of babies? Then hire someone who takes orders well. Or are you a secretly terrified newbie who can't believe she's having one baby, let alone two, and has never even seen a diaper changed? In that case, hire a bossy, experienced coach of a nanny willing to take the helm and teach you everything she knows. Are you super-organized and anticipating weeks of delegating and managing your corps of help? You might get away with a mature teenager. Or are you at this very moment curled up in the fetal position in your closet, praying to St. Jude, Patron Saint of Hopeless Causes? If so, you need to cash in an IRA and find the pricey local legend Mary Poppins–type who can come in and show you how it's done before she pulls away in her Mercedes.

## Interviewing a Potential Nanny

### Topics to cover in an initial phone interview:

- Experience with young children
- Availability
- Criminal record/comfort with background check
- Willingness to get MMR and flu vaccines
- References
- Driver's license? Driving record?
- Current/last work situation
- Willingness to sign a contract
- Willingness to do housework (light)
- Salary requirements

### Questions to ask during a personal interview:

- What is your experience with babies?
- What is your experience with more than one child at a time?
- Have you ever worked with twins?
- Have you ever worked with premature babies?
- What do you like most about children?
- What do you like most about being a nanny?
- What do children like most about you?
- What is most challenging about caring for babies?
- What is most challenging about caring for toddlers?
- Can you elaborate on why you're leaving your previous position?
- Have you ever been faced with an emergency with a child? What happened?
- What do you do when a baby cries?

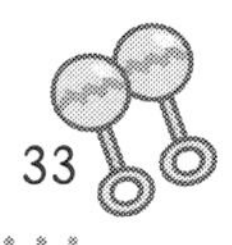

- What is hardest about being a nanny?
- Have you studied child development in a school setting?
- What works best for you when a toddler is having a meltdown?
- Do you smoke?
- What do you tend to prepare for a small child's lunch? Dinner?
- Do you have first aid training and CPR certification? If not, are you willing to get them?
- What do you like to do in your spare time?
- Have you ever disagreed with a parent about the disciplining of his or her child? How did you handle that conflict?
- Describe the best job you ever had.
- How flexible is your schedule? Could you ever work late or on a weekend?
- Do you feel that you have a good sense of what this position requires?
- What questions do you have for us?

## Overnight Nannies

Some moms of twins insist that what is really needed is someone to help during the night. In this case, the primary caretaker can at least string together a decent number of hours of sleep in order to refuel for the next day. The need for nighttime help has created a mini-industry of overnight nannies in many areas of the country, most of whom focus on multiples, but some of whom are hired to keep wealthy parents of singletons well-rested and unpuffy. That's not sour grapes; at the rates they charge, you'd have to be pretty well-off to justify hiring overnight help for a single baby. Whereas there is plenty of work to keep a nanny (or a mommy) hopping all night long with twins, a single baby who sleeps several hours at a time leaves a lot of down time for an overnight nanny.

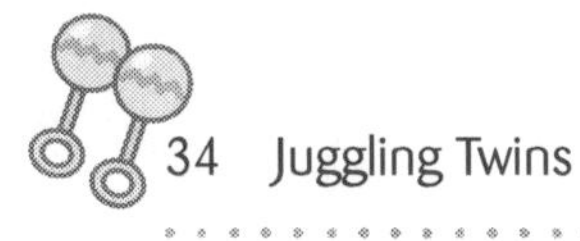


In any case, an overnight nanny is a completely justifiable expense for the parents of twins, though the first time you see the going rates, your knees will buckle and you may hear yourself whimper. Sitting down? At the time of writing of this book, overnight nanny rates where I live range from $250 to $350 per night. Most of us can't afford overnight help *every* night and thus stagger it on intermittent nights, to take the edge off as regularly as possible. In our first weeks, we had someone come three nights a week. By six weeks, we were down to twice a week, and by three months, they were gone. We still miss them.

The function of an overnight baby nurse is to feed, change, settle, and care for the twins all night and in her spare time do any light housekeeping she can manage, including dishes and baby laundry. Generally, they will tidy up the nursery during idle moments. They tend to arrive around 9:00 or 10:00 p.m., at which point the grateful parents hand off their little bundles, traipse off to bed, and collapse until 6:30 a.m. or so, when the shift ends. Arising in the morning, the well-rested couple generally finds dozing, dry, well-fed babies swaddled in a crib or bassinet, a tidy kitchen, and several neat piles of folded clothing on the counter. In a word: order. As they write a big, fat check to hand the nanny on her way out, they feel no regret whatsoever.

It is important to note, particularly if there is some disagreement with your co-parent about the necessity of this expense, that a good night's sleep is a benefit to both of you. Presumably, one of you is headed off to work. It is every bit as difficult to put in a decent day's work on interrupted and depleted sleep as it is to care for babies. Both of you will need a full night's sleep now and then, and you will not be able to ask a neighbor to stay awake all night with your babies. Well, you can try, I suppose. Good luck with that. This is an area of labor that is generally best left to the professionals—you, your partner, and an overnight nanny—though some families do have the good fortune to have competent, willing family members who can occasionally do an overnight shift. Again, an overnight nanny is expensive but can be a lifesaver even if only scheduled for a couple of times per week.

## Reality Check

I nearly cried with relief the first evening the overnight nanny arrived and I knew that I would be able to sleep the entire night through. After all, the sleep deprivation begins well before the babies are born; for me it began as I slept every night of the last few weeks of my pregnancy upright in an overstuffed chair, having found it impossible to sleep in my bed any longer. By the first evening the nanny arrived, I felt as if I had been awake for several years; it was a profound exhaustion such as I had never before felt and haven't since. My cells were tired. Imagine my surprise, then, when the nanny cheerfully reminded me that she would be bringing me the babies one by one to be nursed within a few hours. I was stunned by this betrayal. Yes, I had nursed a child before this. Yes, I had been nursing these babies throughout the nights since they were born. But no, it had not occurred to me that I would still need to feed them myself even though I had expressed milk in the freezer, or would at least need to pump if I didn't want to explode in my sleep. My welling tears of relief turned quickly to real tears of anguish. I just wanted to sleep.

### Nursing Moms

Yes, it still makes sense to hire someone overnight when you are nursing. It doesn't make as *much* sense as it does for those feeding with formula. In that case, it makes beautiful, perfect, absolute sense. Still, for a nursing mom, it makes a big difference. While the nanny did in fact deliver babies to me during the night, there is an enormous difference between having a baby placed next to you in your bed so that she can suckle while you doze, and getting up out of

bed to pick up, feed, burp, change, swaddle, and resettle a baby—at least four times. Even during the weeks when I was working hard at pumping in order to get my milk supply established, I became adept at sleeping in that overstuffed chair as I pumped. Please try not to focus on that image of me—hooked up and passed out—any longer than necessary; just know it can be done. When I was finished, the nanny would collect the milk, whisk the whole thing away, and have the milk stored and the pump cleaned when I awoke. One huge difference in the nights that we had the nanny was that we rarely heard crying. We were off duty, and for once we could turn off the baby radar and let someone else worry about them. That short break from their siren calls might itself have been worth the entire cost.

## Other Considerations

The amount and type of help you need is determined in part by whether or not you have an older child or children. Look at the whole picture of your household in action before settling on someone. Hiring someone who is comfortable only with the older child or only with the babies will limit your options significantly. Because that older child is going to need you more than ever, it helps to find someone who can stay alone with the babies at least long enough for you to read to your older child or drive her to preschool yourself now and then. I know of a woman who was resentful when her nanny played all day with her three-year-old son while she "knocked (herself) out caring for the babies."

I have heard many women say that if they were to do it again, they wouldn't hire child care at all but would instead hire a full-time housekeeper, so that they could focus entirely on the children while someone else did the less appealing work. Now, *that* makes sense to me, and the next time I find a spare stack of hundreds, that's exactly what I plan to do. Perhaps the best solution for you will be an overnight nanny a few nights a week and a teenager for a few afternoons, or some similar combination. Or, like us, you might sign on to two to three nights of help and then rely on friends and family for any day help. Or it may indeed make more sense for you to hire day help, instead. However you decide to pace your funds and arrange your help, bear in mind the basic unfairness of expecting anyone, paid or not, to do what you yourself cannot. She is a nanny, not a superhero.

Whatever your decision at this point, there will surely be some adjustments to the schedule once you have had some time to see how it works or doesn't work, and how your needs are changing. The basic premise, however, is for several months to be able to start every day with the knowledge that at some point, someone will be arriving to help you, if only for an hour so that you can take a shower or a nap. This promise of incoming aid is psychologically important; it's good to have a goal, even if it is as simple as getting out of your pajamas at some point during the week. You may be amazed by the sudden preciousness of formerly simple propositions like a hot shower, a ten-minute break to scan the headlines of the newspaper, or a decent walk with the dog, whose name you can no longer remember without considerable effort. Hopefully, you will be helped by people that you also happen to like and who also happen to like your kids. Not only will the adult company and conversation be refreshing, but another caretaker will also be more willing than most of your friends to work through with you all the obsessive observations and questions you have about your babies. If you're really lucky, they'll have some answers, too.

# 5

# Organizing the Household

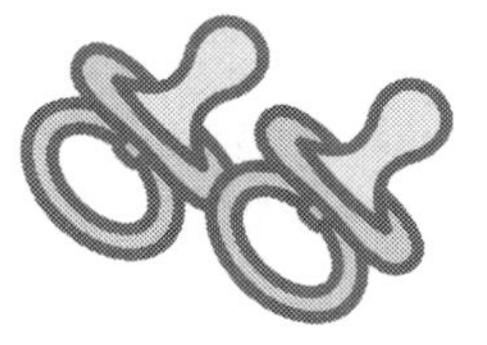

Think of the Home with Newborn Twins as a manufacturing plant. Stay with me here, and I promise not to shatter your romantic-love-fest-baby-nirvana-vision thing entirely. It's a factory with three divisions of labor: there's the obvious and newly launched Department of Baby Management. There's also the longstanding Household Maintenance Department and for some, a third division of industry, the Older Sibling Preservation Department.

Within the large arm of the Household Maintenance Department, there are two divisions: Immediate Concerns and Long-Term Projects...the latter of which has been temporarily mothballed, because there will be no painting projects, kitchen renovations, or gutter-cleaning assignments for at least a few months. Maintenance now refers simply to the removal of objects from the floor, the straightening of clutter, the wiping of counters, and the washing of dishes and laundry. Note that bed making, dusting, and even vacuuming do not necessarily make this stripped-down list on a daily basis. They are luxuries that are only attempted if the maintenance department inadvertently schedules too many laborers one day.

If you have an Older Sibling Preservation Department, you may have noticed that he, she, or they have their own demands. They still have some inexplicable expectation of being fed, dressed, spoken to, and occasionally played with. And while it's not on *their* wish list, a bath now and then would be good, too. Now, while the polite thing for them to do—the true team-player approach—would be to suck it up, demand less attention for a while, and exercise a *little* self-sufficiency for once, it is pretty well established that it is at this point that an older sibling suddenly has a justifiably ravenous appetite for attention. So this department will be in full swing for a while.

It seems to be the natural succession of power that the bearer of the twins is the de facto CEO of this factory. As such, you need to get as much of the organization of labor accomplished ahead of the actual shifts as is possible. As we discussed in the previous chapter, the scheduling of helpers, both volunteer and paid, should happen by your third trimester and should be detailed, cemented, and written on a master calendar. Obviously, there will be some room for amendments as you go, but at the very least, you need to have a preliminary plan from the get-go. In particular, be sure that those first weeks are mapped out carefully as to who will be staying with you and who will be visiting (to help, not to chat or ogle) in the short term. While some moms claim that after the births, they just couldn't wait to get out of the hospital and start life with their newborns, others of us absolutely savor the postpartum five hours or so that insurance companies now allow new moms to stay on the maternity ward. Okay, maybe it's 48...in any case, it's an absurdly short time before they now hand you your hat and your kids and show you the door...and no, they don't double it for twins.

If you are at all like me, you will experience extreme reluctance to leave the maternity ward, where those unbelievably competent and reassuring nurses have helped you to get the babies to latch on, whisked them away when you were fatigued, brought you the cup of coffee that you have been waiting for nine months to sip, and taught you to swaddle the babies like little origami burritos. You will in fact grow so quickly accustomed to being pampered that you will begin complaining of nonexistent symptoms and willing your blood pressure to escalate precipitously in order to extend your stay. Whether your emergence from the maternity ward is voluntary or

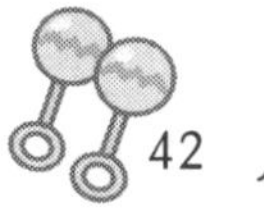



involves the application of a nurse's clog-encased foot to your rear end, your arrival home will be even more wonderful and you will be much better able to appreciate its momentousness if the help is previously scheduled and the shifts have already begun when you make that first trip through the door.

## Get Started Now

Beyond organizing the labor force, a number of tasks can and should be completed while you are gestating. With a singleton pregnancy, I would encourage you to get through a to-do list during the third trimester. But with multiples, it's never smart to count on the third trimester as a productive time. While some of us manage to go nearly fully to term, there is a decent chance that you could end up on bed rest at some point—a point most likely to happen during the third trimester—or that the babies might make their appearance during what you assumed would be the last part of your pregnancy. Don't count on the last two months as your own. If you get them and they are even remotely productive for you, that's a bonus, as you are also going to be tired in a manner that you've never experienced before. Therefore, you want to work your way through the following suggestions somewhere between the moment when you have decided the pregnancy is real and the moment when you are too incapacitated to accomplish anything. That window occupies about a week in the middle of your second trimester. When you recognize it, pounce.

### Meal Planning: Freeze Now, Eat Later

Primary on your list are endeavors we have already discussed, including the planning of the diaper party and the scheduling of the volunteer corps and their paid counterparts. The third item on your list is some advance planning on meals. While it may already have occurred to you that an inordinate amount of time in a typical household is dedicated to the planning, purchasing, and preparing of meals and the recurring, onerous cleanup thereafter, the unremitting need of my family to *eat yet again* never fails to take me by surprise. I will remember these years primarily as the ones during which I stood in front of the open fridge and freezer an hour before every meal saying, "Hmmm." Every mealtime makes me wonder, "Didn't we just do this?" and this is the real reason I like brunch: it eliminates one of those moments of wondering what to feed everyone.

The sort of time that whole process requires won't be available to you in the first weeks with twins, and it's better not to tie up your help in the creation of five-star meals, either. The more you can make and freeze now, the better. Yes, you will be able to order in; yes, friends will arrive with meals; and yes, you can always resort to dining on cereal and milk now and then. But it is really great to have a freezer stocked with healthy ready-to-go meals that you know you like. We made the mistake of making loads of lasagna, forgetting that upwards of 83 percent of meals that friends and neighbors bring in after a birth are lasagna or lasagna-like. Suffice it to say I'm unlikely to touch the stuff again before our twins are in graduate school. Better to go with soups and stews, burritos preassembled and individually wrapped, pot pies, and chili (easy on the beans and onions if you're going to nurse). Throw five or ten decent baguettes in there, too. Stuff the freezer with as many entrees as it will hold so that it's possible to grab an entrée, nuke it, throw a bagged salad in a bowl and a loaf of bread in the oven to warm, and voilà! Dinner in ten minutes. I've known some parents of twins who went so far as to use paper plates and plastic utensils for a number of weeks, and while the environmentalist in me says that's going too far, the environmentalist in you may have her mouth duct-taped by the survivor in you at this very moment.

For us, the preparation of these frozen meals happened only after a giant warehouse-store run. Not only did we stock up on frozen chicken breasts, butter, fruit, seafood, coffee beans, and pretty much anything that could be kept at 0 degrees indefinitely, but we also supplied our house like a fallout shelter with everything from mouthwash to number two pencils. Those who are convinced that a pandemic flu is inevitable could have taken a lesson from our approach; basically, we stocked the house such that the only reason to go to the grocery store when the babies were infants was for emergency cilantro or more milk. This trip, which quite literally cost us more than I spent on my first car, may be for you one of the first moments of realizing that this twin project is an expensive proposition. As with the hiring of help, there are indeed elements of these months that may be more costly than, say, any previous month of your life. But these expenses do in fact taper off (until the kids are in college, but let's not go there). Buying in bulk ends up being a cost-saver if you can manage the initial output, just as ponying up for help during those first months will save your sanity.

## Birth Announcements

Another task that can be accomplished while you are still *with children* is to choose the design of your birth announcement and get as far along in that process as is possible without an actual birth. Minimally, you can address all the envelopes and get the stamps on them. If you are designing your own announcement online, you can pretty much do everything but add names and weights and hit "send." If you're really trying to get a jump on things and know the kids' names already, why not just throw an average weight and a probable date on the thing and check it right off that list? Efficiency, efficiency! More practically, you can at this point buy dozens of thank-you cards and plenty of stamps. Make no mistake, though: the writing of thank-you cards should eventually become your partner's responsibility. Feel free to highlight this as textual evidence of the obvious…I mean, really, after you carried them all those months, you deserve a pass on this one even if it's normally in your domestic jurisdiction.

## Baby Station Setup

Before the births are imminent, it is a good idea to set up the areas where the babies will be hanging out in the first months. If you have a house or apartment that occupies one floor, you have half the work of those who have two. If your home has two floors, you absolutely want to set up not just the nursery but also a second baby station downstairs. If the notion of using your living room as a nursery doesn't appeal to your sense of interior design, suck it up. This is a temporary setup, and within a few months you can sequester these children as far from your Pottery Barn ensemble as you wish. For the immediate future, however, you will appreciate having the babies in the center of your home, rather than in their room, and mostly you will appreciate not taking 400 trips up the stairs daily, both with and without babies in your arms. If you are able to create a space that can be darkened with heavy drapes, closed off with doors, and air conditioned in the hot months, you're looking at the perfect baby station. If not, bear in mind that newborn babies can sleep with light, with noise, and with fans. A living room not too far from the kitchen or a formal dining room that doesn't get daily use would be perfect, but the truth is that any room will do. At the beginning, you only need the following items in this room:

- One crib with appropriate bedding and bumpers and perhaps two of those cool, foam wedge doohickeys that help babies stay on their backs. The babies will happily share one crib in the beginning (more on that below).

- A diapering station with a changing pad, wipes, diapers (aka dipes), and a dipe receptacle if you can stand having it in your living room (eventually we used the plastic bags from our delivered newspapers, twisted them up and threw them right in our kitchen trash, rather than have a Diaper Champ as an end table). Notice you *do not need a changing table* in your living room, just a surface around two to four feet high on which you can put the pad. We have never had a changing table, even in our kids' nurseries. Short dressers work fine and the top drawer holds everything we need.

- A couple of chairs or a sofa on which feeders of babies can sit.

That's it! Now you have a place where the babies can be jiggled, changed, fed, and put down to sleep that's not off in another wing of the house. This makes the transferring of baby duties easier, the answering of a telephone now and then more likely, and the chance of your feeling isolated in the nursery for weeks on end remote. The babies can spend their day downstairs and then you can bring them upstairs with you to their nursery or to your room when you head off to bed. On a blessed night when some hired angel will be arriving to care for your babies, she can care for them in their downstairs satellite station, out of your private quarters, out of your earshot, and close to any light household chores she is able to attack. If she needs to bring you a baby, she can knock politely on your bedroom door.

With or without a second floor, you are likely to be setting up a nursery for these babies. One crib will suffice at the beginning.[1] Our babies actually shared one cradle for weeks. Many twin specialists believe that twins need regular proximity to their cohorts, having been smooshed together for months and having grown used to the heartbeat of the other. I was so moved by that idea when I read it

---

1. The exact benefits and risks of "co-bedding" twins are not clearly established yet, though there has been much attention given to this practice in medical research in the past decade. While most NICUs, for example, tend in practice to co-bed their preemie twins in order to regulate their heartbeats, some researchers suggest the possibility that the presence of another baby in the crib may increase the likelihood of SIDS. Please research this question to your own satisfaction before deciding whether or not to put your babies down in the same crib. Your decision may depend upon your circumstances; i.e., you may be more comfortable doing so if there is a night nurse with the babies. Regardless of where they sleep, remember that babies must sleep on their backs.

while pregnant that I endeavored always to have them sleep close together at the beginning. Admittedly, I was disappointed by their seemingly total disregard for one another, but that doesn't mean they didn't benefit at some level by being snuggled next to each other routinely. My feeling, however, is that all babies need a sense of containment in order to be settled, and that two singleton infants would probably enjoy spooning, too. Who wouldn't? In the end, though, swaddling our babies did more to make them feel comfortable than did enforcing their togetherness. It took them several months even to look over at each other and wonder, "Who are you, and what are you doing in my crib?" Their utter self-centeredness did give way to an intensely close relationship when they grew a bit, so there's no need to decide your children don't like one another just because they don't curl up together like piglets at the beginning.

## Hospital and Visitation Rules

We take for granted some of the age-old traditions around welcoming new babies, but they don't all work well for an exhausted family that is adjusting to *two* brand-new infants. Abandoning some of these welcoming traditions is an important step in getting off to a sane and rested start with your babies. When the woman who runs a local overnight nanny service in our area urged us to issue a set of draconian rules about hospital visitations and procedures, I was a bit put off, having really enjoyed the postpartum party scene in my eldest's birthing room. "What?" I thought. "No champagne? No gaggles of friends bearing Kung Pao chicken?" But she was tough on this issue and was, as always, correct. Whereas life with one newborn starts with reaching out, life with two newborns begins with hunkering down. Here are her rules. Feel free to issue them to friends and family sometime during your third trimester:

1. No visitors at the hospital. None. Your time there is very limited, and you need every minute of it not simply to eat, rest, and recover before coming home to a challenging situation, but also to go to

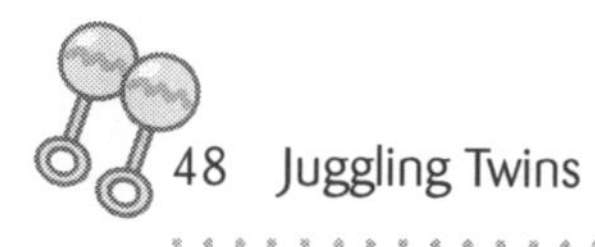


every breastfeeding course, to get used to holding both babies at once, and to practice swaddling and latching on in the company of nurse experts.

2. Ditto for phone calls.

3. No gifts at the hospital. Have all flowers, stuffed animals, and balloons sent to your home. It's hard enough carrying two babies along with all the stuff you will be stealing...which leads to...

4. Pilfer pitilessly. Don't *steal*. That's wrong, as you are probably aware. But do take advantage of every handout or promotional gift that comes your way and be sure to ask if there are any more available. Abandon your manners entirely.

## Free Loot at the Hospital

Even if you plan to nurse, hoard all the free formula they give you, and then casually suggest that you might need more. Worst-case scenario: it will save you a trip to the store if you run out of half and half for your coffee one day. Make a special effort to collect and bring home all the tiny little two-ounce "disposable" bottles they have for newborns, because, guess what? They wash up just fine and are great for the early weeks. Those perfectly sized little T-shirts that have coverings over the hands so that the baby can't gouge her own eyeballs? Beg your nurse for them. The pacifiers they use? Ooops... they keep falling into your duffel bag. (They're disposable; you are not robbing some other baby, I promise.)

Our mentor's advice—which was absolutely right—also extended beyond the hospital stay, as she elicited promises from us to limit visitors to fifteen-minute stays and not to allow germy children (all those between 1–17 years) on the premises in the first weeks. Those were, admittedly, tough ones to keep. We loved having visitors gawk and coo at the babies and spend time with our five-year-old, and some of our favorite visitors were children, whose wide-eyed amazement at the twins mirrored our own feelings precisely. In the first weeks, though, it is a better idea to send everyone digital photos and ask them to hold off on visits.

Below is a brief recap of what you need to focus on before you are too large to focus on anything but your own immensity.

## To-Do List: Third Trimester

- ☐ Organize the help schedule.
- ☐ Make a warehouse-store run/freeze meals.
- ☐ Prepare announcements and thank-you notes.
- ☐ Set up babies' stations.
- ☐ Issue hospital and early visitation rules.
- ☐ Shop/troll for equipment basics.

# 6

# The Stuff: What You'll Really Need

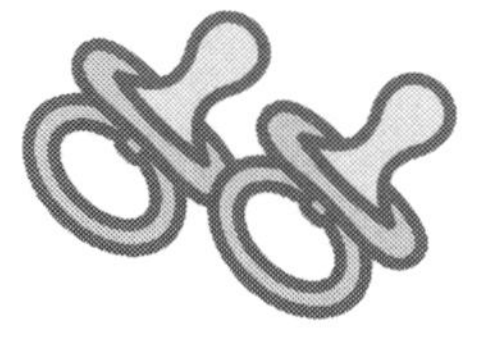

By now you have perhaps observed that *economy* is the theme that should run through this entire endeavor—not just your allotment of time when caring for twins, but also your allotment of funds for the long haul. In that spirit, I suggest that you forage for used equipment before you shop for or "wish list" the new stuff. Below are three lists that can help you decide what items are most important:

## A List: Items You Truly Need, and Should Probably Have When the Babies Come Home

*Don't be surprised if friends and family supply your entire A List, assuming you are savvy enough to make it a public document.*

### Clothes

- At least 10 infant gowns
- 2 homecoming outfits, if you must
- 12–16 onesie shirts, including 2–4 with hand coverings
- 2 hats
- 4 pairs socks
- For winter babies, add:
  - 4 sweaters or warm shirts
  - 2 Bundle Me bunting sets (or similar)

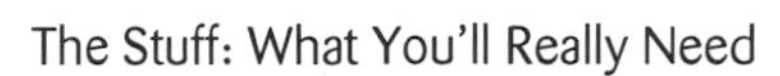

### Gear

- 2 infant car seats
- 2 bouncy seats for each floor of the house
- 1 sling/baby carrier (such as Baby Bjorn)

### Diapering

- Case of diapers (You can get these for free! See page 12)
- Wipes
- A tub of a zinc oxide–based diaper cream

### Nursery

- 1 crib with mattress for each floor of house
- Bumpers/2 mattress pads and 2 sheets for each crib
- At least 6 swaddling blankets
- 12 flat cotton diapers to use as burp cloths
- Changing pad and cover for each floor of house
- Baby monitor
- Glider or rocker
- Ottoman or nursing stool

### Baby Care

- 4 newborn pacifiers (try various brands)
- Nail scissors
- Thermometer
- Baby wash

### Feeding

- 6–8 bottles and nipples
- Can of powdered formula

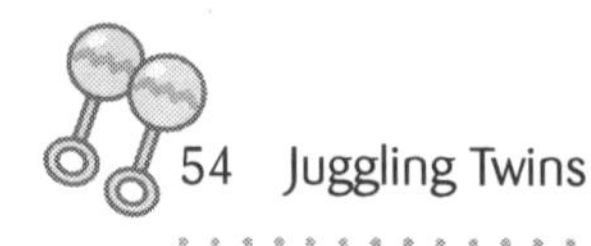


- Bottle brush
- If breastfeeding:
  - Twin nursing pillow
  - Box of breast pads

Infant gowns are those over-the-head shirts that extend well beyond the length of the child and have elastic at the bottom to cinch the tot contents like a little bag of potatoes. They create a "bag-o'-baby" effect. These are pretty much what my kids lived in for the first few months. There is nothing more stupid than pants for babies. Not only do they not flatter the newborn figure, but they are a total pain for the diaper changer to wrangle with. With the gowns, one simply places the baby on a table and slides the thing up. Instant access. They are big enough for those little legs to pedal and kick all they need to, and they are pretty cute, too. Yes, for boys, too. We had a pile of about a dozen of them and that, plus the infant T-shirts, were all our kids wore for a very long time. (We had pretty much cashed in all those 0–3 month clothes by now anyway and had stuffed the proceeds into the college fund.)

Another crucial A-List component: bouncy seats, two on each floor of your house. You need some baby repositories, and bouncy seats are great because they keep kids contained and safe. Most of them now have a "vibrate" feature as well, which for some squawking newborns can bring miraculous peace. Bouncy seats are portable and can be moved easily, with sleeping baby aboard, from floor to dining room table to kitchen as needed. While they are designed for slightly older kids, we strapped tightly swaddled newborns in them and found that they were quite content and totally stable. The key is that the swaddle keeps the baby from moving around and tipping while in the bouncy seat. You should *never* place a newborn in a bouncy seat without a tight swaddle.

The bouncy seats are also pitched at the perfect angle for just-fed or congested babies who might be less comfortable when prone. Our bouncy seats were indispensable to us, and we used them until the kids were so big that the back of the thing swayed low under their weight and the boys could unbuckle them, get up, and walk away. As with most of these devices, the used ones work fine. The cloth covers are washable, and you don't need to get all the bells and whistles of musical/light/mobile combinations that will only make your child feel she's being raised in a video arcade.

Please note that there's no mention of an expensive breast pump on List A; this big-ticket item is relegated to List B. Even if you are absolutely resolute about breastfeeding, you should hold off before plunking down a few hundred dollars on a breast pump that disguises itself as a groovy briefcase and stores more chilled milk than you could pump on a three-week vacation. If you can borrow a breast pump, by all means do. The companies that produce them issue warnings about using others' breast pumps that are clearly designed to frighten fragile mothers into thinking that they will be poisoning their babies with others' bacteria-ridden milky residue. As far as I'm concerned, this is simply a marketing strategy. These units are built to be sterilized, and if they weren't, the original owner's baby would also be sick. Every piece comes off and can and should be boiled relentlessly or replaced and is then good to go.

I lent my pump to four different friends and used it for a couple of years myself, and it's still going strong, and so are all of the five children who drank the milk it pumped. This is a very expensive item, so hunt around for a friend's or get on the Internet and find a used one if you can. But don't feel that you need to have this taken care of by your third trimester. You won't be pumping to get supply up until breastfeeding is fairly well established, and even if your babies were to come early, you would have access to good pumps through the hospital and may want to weigh rental options.

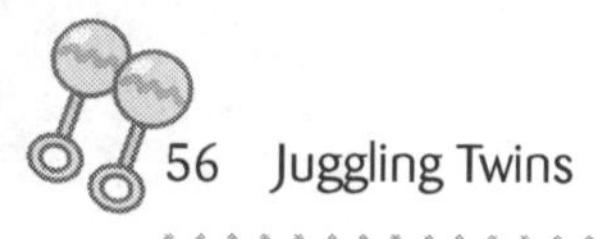


## B List: Items That You Will Eventually Need

*These are the things that you should wait to purchase, because they are likely baby gifts. None is immediately necessary, so wait and see what the UPS driver brings and then fill in later where you feel you must. They are listed in order of probable need over time.*

- Breast pump
- Double stroller
- Swing
- 2 portable cribs (e.g., Pack-n-Play) and sheets
- Another sling/baby carrier (e.g., Baby Bjorn)
- Diaper bag
- Diaper depository and liners
- 2 bulb syringes
- Bathtub
- Nursery décor (e.g., curtains, lamps, pictures)
- Humidifier/vaporizer
- Brush and comb
- 2 car baby mirrors
- 2 mobiles
- First-aid supplies
- Dishwasher caddy
- Drying rack
- Hooded baby towels
- Playmat and "gym" or play arch
- Lullaby and baby music
- Eventually, another crib
- Doorway jumper seats
- An exersaucer or stationary play center (or 2)

There is a lot of debate about which type of stroller is the best to buy, and because it is a big-ticket item, it is worth putting some time into your own investigation. The basic decision is between side-by-side and tandem models, and the central arguments are that side-by-sides fold smaller and are maneuverable but tandems fit better through doors and store aisles. Unless you plan to take your newborns out for a stroll the first day you get home, a stroller is not an immediate need. When the babies are tiny, you will transport them in two car seats from the house to the car and the car to the pediatrician's office. You won't be able to do so for too long, though, and will eventually need a stroller.

The limousine of twin infant transport is the stadium-seating, three-wheeled frame that holds two infant car seats. The original version was called a Double Decker and it is hugely popular with parents of twins as it allows them to move sleeping babies between stroller and car, it is amazingly maneuverable, and the babies have equal access to a decent view. It is pricey, but many feel it is worth it, particularly if you can find a used one or resell yours later. Once the babies are out of their infant seats, it is useless, and this happens blindingly quickly. There are many models, however, that are suitable for both infants and toddlers, so put some time into researching this question. We have had both cheap strollers and pricey ones, and I must say that they all break eventually, including those that required a second mortgage to purchase. Our solution was to pick up a friend's ten-year-old umbrella side-by-side that was already well worn and use it for travel, so that we didn't have to worry about having it bounce down tarmacs or get crushed in our car carrier. We bought a more expensive one, but it stayed home during trips. We used it almost daily until the kids were about three years old.

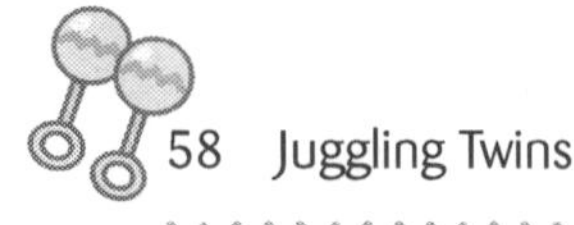


There are now some very cool double baby joggers on the market that are basically all-terrain vehicles that have adjustable suspension and are totally maneuverable. Sometimes people even jog with them! We had one that we used only for actual jogging with babies, as ours was outdated and didn't fold easily to put into the car. Joggers are a great supplementary item, but if your budget doesn't allow for both, the stroller is probably the one to choose.

One swing is probably enough. These contraptions are marvels for lulling little ones to sleep and can be a great way to keep one baby happy while you are dealing with the other. They take up a huge amount of floor space, however, and the number of times that you would actually pop two babies into swings simultaneously is small enough that the expense isn't justifiable. You will, however, eventually need two portable cribs (aka Pack-n-Plays) if you and your babies ever want to leave your house for more than a day. These can double as playpens and can hold kids three years later if, for example, you want a strep-ridden, nauseated toddler to sleep in your room but not on you, or you want to separate your kids at naptime. Buying two of these *is* a justifiable expense, but they are durable, so consider buying them used. When our twins were three months old, we took them on their first camping trip, and we actually set up a Pack-n-Play in a tent for them. They were happy as can be, and we were wishing we had similar accommodations for the rest of us.

While you definitely want one Baby Bjorn or an equivalent waiting for you when you get home from the hospital, it's not crucial that you have a second one immediately. A co-parent or helper can comfort a baby in one while you deal with the other. In time, though, it's nice for each of you to be able to carry a baby on a stroll or shopping trip and have your hands free. More importantly, babies love them and are comforted by their closeness to the person carrying them. One of our sons really loved his and seemed to feel safest in it; it was the one sure comfort for him when he was out of sorts, and he spent many early evening hours riding happily on the nearest available adult.

For our first child, we had an elaborate diaper bag. With the twins, we used one of our old hiking day packs and loved it. It had more space and pockets, as well as two shoulder straps, which prevented our doing the "purse pinch," whereby one awkwardly holds one shoulder close to the ear to keep the bag's strap in place. It also reminded us nostalgically of our former life, when we actually hiked. You may already own a day pack that will serve easily as a diaper bag, and you will probably find that a dad is much more willing to carry it than he would be to carry a pink and green Lilly Pulitzer diaper bag. You also don't need to go out immediately to buy one of those funky-looking bulb aspirators used to vacuum mucus out of baby noses. Be assured the hospital will not want to take back the one they have been using on your child and will send it home with you along with all the other little door prizes they now give their lucky contestants.

As for diaper receptacles, we were converted as former disciples of the Diaper Genie, which makes a diaper-sausage out of a long string of used dipes, to the Diaper Champ, which has a top that clamps down but flips over, so that dirty diapers are delivered into a kitchen trash bag below. The Champ involves less labor and less odor. Either way, you are bound to feel extraordinary guilt for the pile of diapers you will be adding to landfills in the next few years. It is an astonishing number. If you have the stomach and the budget for a diaper delivery service, more power to you, my green friend.

There are now all sorts of plastic baby holders for the bathtub, and we had several, including the recliner seats with foam on the bottom and the rings they sit in when they can sit up. Interestingly, though, whenever our expert night nannies bathed the kids, they did so in the kitchen sink, which they thought safer because they themselves were on their feet, rather than kneeling and reaching. It may be that you don't need bath furniture at all.

One of the final items on the B List is jumpy seats, which are suspended seats that hook solidly to the top of a door frame and allow your kids to propel themselves like bungee jumpers with Flubber on their feet. We loved them but were reprimanded well into our love affair by a friend who is a chiropractor and claimed they were unhealthy for developing baby legs. Ours made it through the experience with fully functioning legs, but who am I to say if that was just lucky? They are a wonderfully entertaining depository for older babies, but perhaps you will not want to risk their limbs in the way that we apparently did.

## F List: Keep the Tags On; It's Going Back

*The last list itemizes your personal "returns" bin. Think of these silly, useless, redundant, or simply offensive items as chits to trade in for money for formula.*

- Infant shoes (Think about it.)
- Baby washcloths (As it turns out, yours work on babies, too.)
- Bottle "carriers" (They've been transported for years without them.)
- Bottle warmers (A pan of warm water holds two bottles and works perfectly.)
- Pacifier holders (Puh-lease!)
- Grocery cart seat covers (Let the kid build a *little* immunity.)
- Diaper stackers (Diapers aren't very unruly; you can handle them.)

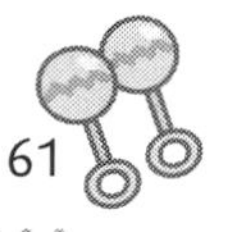

- Wipe warmers (Do you want to raise sissies? When I was a kid, they used leftover sandpaper. Builds moral character.)
- Walkers (Danger, Will Robinson! They tend to catapult their infant drivers down the stairs.)

Eventually, you are going to need all manner of babyproofing locks, guards and pads, some bibs, a couple of high chairs, gates, toilet-seat rings, toddler-bed guards, car-window shades, nightlights, blanket sleepers, extra bottles and faster-flowing nipples, rubber-tipped spoons and plastic bowls...oh yeah, and maybe a few toys for the poor kids. For the moment, however, pace yourself. You've got more immediate concerns, and shopping for these items may be your excuse to get out of the house a year from now. You're going to need one.

# 7

# To Minivan or Not to Minivan?

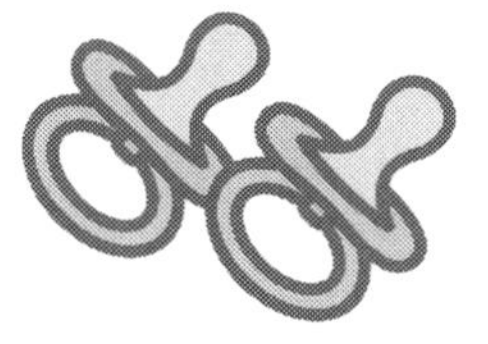

There is a certain pathetic resignation in the face of a man behind the wheel of a minivan, whether or not he's being pelted with spit balls by his passengers as he listens to Raffi. Even alone behind the wheel, a man looks beaten. Automobile manufacturers and marketers clearly know that men are a lost cause when it comes to minivans. Their preferred target? The American Mom. But not all of us go down without a good fight. And some of us remain standing.

When we had one toddler and a dog or two, we were perfectly happy in our Subaru station wagon. It had all-wheel drive, good gas mileage, and a more gutsy than suburban look and feel. It didn't advertise our status as parents; in fact, we owned it well before we considered having any children. However, once the ultrasound confirmed that we would be increasing our number of car seats by 200 percent, we knew that the days of our rugged outdoorsy car were limited, because even if the three car seats could fit in the back seat (they couldn't, but can in some cars), we would have broken our backs getting the big kid into the middle seat, or she would have been climbing over the babies in her big rain boots, placing her hands squarely on their heads to balance herself as she passed, in order to get to the middle seat. Either way, there would have been great weeping and gnashing of teeth—perhaps the kids', but more likely, ours.

If your twins are not your first children, you may also be faced with this difficulty, and if you have a dog or dogs, you certainly are, as it is a ridiculous truth that many, many car purchasing decisions are in the end based on our dogs' travel requirements. Even if you are canine-free and your twins are your first children, you may be in the process of realizing that while your trusty Civic may hold two parents and two babies in car seats, you will then only be allowed one carry-on piece each for the trunk. You may be happy having a permanent plastic storage box on top of the car for strollers, Pack-n-Plays, and bouncy seats for Grandma's house, or you may instead decide that you are entering a new era in need of a new ride, because even fitting groceries and a double stroller in a standard trunk can be challenging, especially once you see how much more food you're buying.

Once you step over, even gingerly, into the Land of Car Shopping, the siren call of the minivan will purr its enchanting melody to you. Whereas these ubiquitous boxes-on-wheels in their muted silvers and sand-tones were invisible to you only last year, now you will recognize that you are completely surrounded by them, and when you inquire, their satisfied owners will begin with a zealot's fervor to extol the glory of their conveniences. These vehicles are, after all, built with you in mind. Their doors open automatically as you approach them with your arms full of children. The manufacturers have placed a DVD player four inches before the nose of each child in order to assure you of his or her entranced compliance over multiple sixteen-hour trips. Each seat has three or four cup holders next to it to help stave off what increasingly appears to be a national dehydration epidemic. The back well seems to have been carved perfectly to cradle a stroller, and the seats fold like origami into any position you can imagine so that pretty much any configuration of big people/small people/animals/equipment will fit and can be arranged without a bead of sweat ever forming on your brow.

On the verge of signing the sales agreement for one of these kid-toting machines, I sat in the driver's seat, seven months pregnant

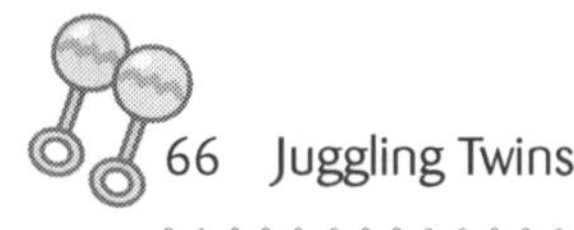


and barely able to reach the steering wheel ("No problem, ma'am, we can adjust it in thirty-five different positions..."), steeling myself before taking the leap into this ultimate expression of suburban parenthood. I played with the dials of the multi-disc CD player that could pipe "Peter, Paul, and Mommy" to the back row while I listened to Dave Matthews up front. Next to me in the passenger seat was a very sweet twenty-four-year-old salesman whose fingers were already twitching their readiness to count his sales commission. This one was clearly in the bag for him.

And then, something in me snapped with a nearly audible *pfffft!* It may actually have been caused by my stockings' doing that window-shade trick they have during the third trimester, when they roll from just under your breasts to mid-thigh in a nanosecond. In any case, suddenly, I couldn't do it.

"No," I said. "No."

"Sorry, ma'am?"

"No."

"Umm. 'No' what?"

"I can't do this."

"Do what?"

"Buy this. I can't buy this." I turned to his baby face, trying to explain something he was fifteen years from even beginning to understand. "If I buy this car, I am done. Done with hip. Done with my youth. Done with *me*. Done."

"Let me show you the cup holders again."

"No."

"Okay, then what I would like to do is talk about the titanium rods that surround each child to form a protective barrier—"

"I don't care."

"Ma'am?"

"I don't care. My parents took me home from the hospital in a picnic basket on the floor of their Fairlane. I don't care. I'll drive more carefully. I'll stay off the highway entirely. Drive only back roads. But I can't buy this."

He made a last-ditch attempt to convince me that a leather interior would easily offset the mid-life crisis being engendered by this sale, but this was met only by a rise in the volume of my protests, and after I explained that, additionally, his *ma'am*ing me through the process had perhaps deepened my distress, his fingers stopped twitching, the sales commission slipping through them, and he politely excused himself to go hunt for more promising prey in the showroom. He was a nice boy, and I still regret having pulled him so intimately into my struggle with my own mortality, but it is one that he has probably by now been forced to witness more of and perhaps has even come to expect now and then. While the minivan may threaten the masculinity of the American male, its threat for some American females is the destruction of our very fragile grasp on the remaining gossamer threads of our youth. More simply, it threatens full groovicide.

The SUV we bought the next morning has only one cup holder per person, which is actually more than we need, because I never allow children to drink anything on car trips anyway (in fact, I usually start the process of drying them out like little prunes the day before, in order to guarantee bathroom breaks only during gas-ups). It has a third row for the big sister, but in order to get in it, she has to scramble over its seat back, entering from the back hatch, which, until she was seven, I had to open for her. The car apparently does not even know how to open itself and thus requires human manipulation. Its seats slide up and back a few inches but don't pop out, turn around, or convert to billiard tables. It doesn't have one video screen of any sort. When we travel somewhere that we're staying more than, say, twenty minutes, we have to throw baby equipment in the plastic cargo case that has become a nearly permanent fixture on top of the car.

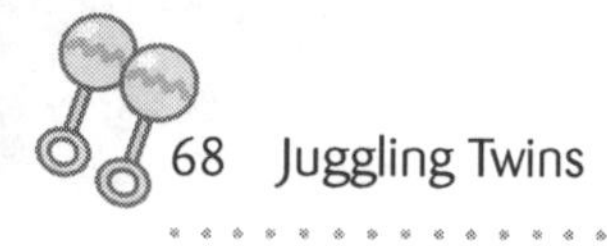


And I am okay with all of that. In fact, I love our car, simply because Mama's still got a fraction of her groove on. It's not a big fraction, but it wouldn't be there at all if I were driving a putty-colored box around town. At some point, a gal's got to draw a line in the sand at the Mortality Beach, and the minivan was where my toe dug deep and traced a fat one. It may be that you are more at peace with the onset of your middle years and the ebbing of your groove, in which case, there's a nice young man whose card I can give you, still out there somewhere trying to meet his monthly minivan sale goal. However, if like me you still cling pitifully to the gossamer threads of your youth, you should know that you can get your kids where they need to go in almost any car with two seat belts in the back. Hold on for all you're worth.

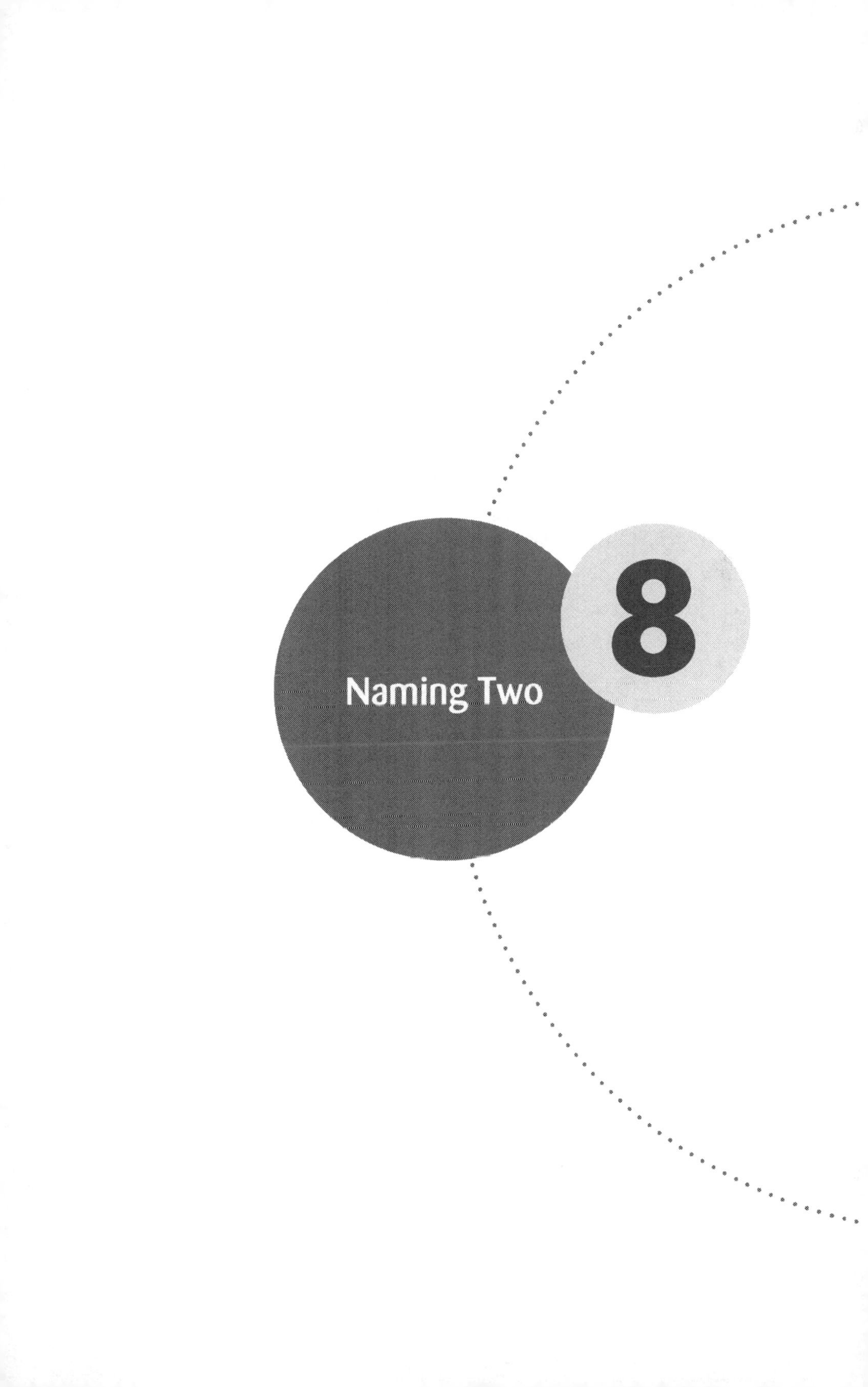
8
Naming Two

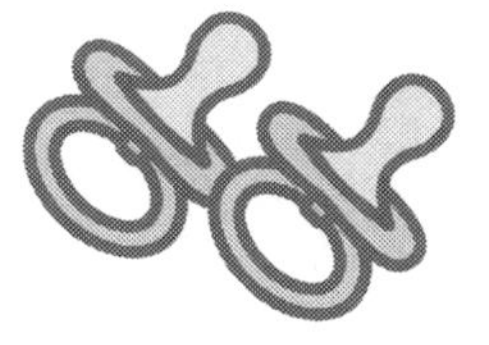

There's a pretty good chance that you already know not only the number of your babies, but also their sexes, and that you can get to work on this naming business early. While I still like being surprised by friends' birth announcements, so many people now not only tell friends if the baby is a boy or girl, but also start using names before the baby has finished growing toes. I'm oddly unnerved by this practice (as in, "Ooooh, Connor has the hiccups today..."). I guess I like the mystery of just thinking of babies in utero as sacred bundles of potentiality, rather than as established little people. I suppose, however, that this tendency to assign names early on is nice in that it begins to establish personhood, and any jump you can get on individuation with twins is great, as they will in some senses be swimming against the tide of their coupledom forever.

In that vein, think carefully about how you name these babies. I trust that you are kind enough and wise enough not to name your babies Frick and Frack, Samson and Deliliah, or Tom and Jerry, but there are subtler traps to fall into, as well. While Romulus and Remus might not have made your short list, you may have to admit to gravitating toward names that rhyme (Matt and Nat, Holly and Molly, or Jack and Zach) or—and this is probably the most common temptation—names that start with the same letter. My mother-in-law, Jan, has a twin sister named Joyce. While I know Joyce very well and spend a good deal of time with her, I often call her "Jan" by mistake. The problem is not their similarity; the problem is the letter *J*.

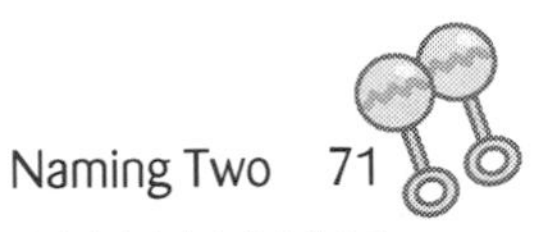

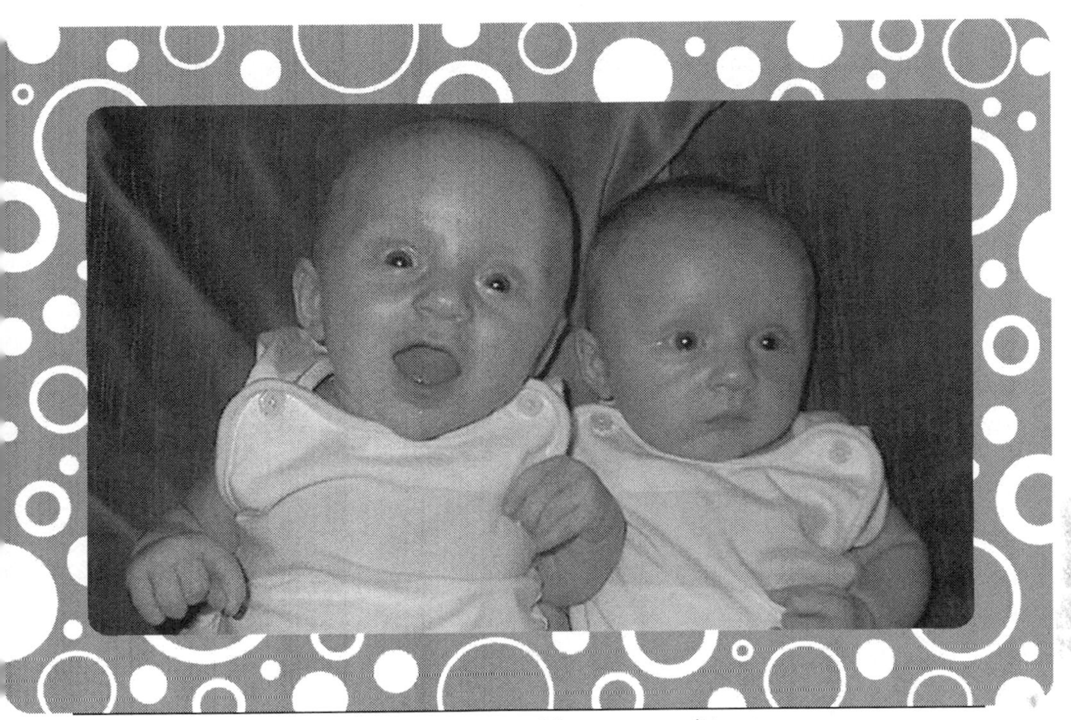

Even identical twins can demonstrate different personalities at a young age.

Photo courtesy of the Regan-Loomis family

If you have other children or pets, you probably already do this regardless of the sounds of their names, and you don't yet have kids who are the same size, possibly with the same face, running around. Tell the truth. Have you *never* yelled at the dog using your spouse's name? I promise you that even if you name your kids Rufus and Calliope, you will still occasionally use the wrong name in your rush to get them out the door for the school bus or to stop one from swinging a seven iron across the back of the other's head. You will make this natural confusion much greater by using names that are at all alike, including the first letter.

Moreover, if it's going to be difficult for *you* to keep them straight, imagine how others will feel. While your twins' close friends will, like your family, eventually roll their eyes when casual acquaintances confuse either them or their names, it is worth noting that over time

we have more casual acquaintances than we do friends and family. The closer the names sound to one another, the more likely your kids are to be called incessantly by the wrong name—particularly if they are identical, but not only in that case. Parents of fraternal twins tell me the problem is not limited to those who look alike; it seems to be a matter of association as much as it is one of truly not being able to see their differences. If the names themselves are similar, they won't get uttered much at all, because people will become even more fearful of getting it wrong and will instead resort to "Hey, how's it going?" or worse, calling them both "Twin" or using their last name to address them. Name your twins just as you would name siblings born years apart...unless you are that family that has a Jessica, Justin, Jacob, Julia, and Joshua.

## Reality Check

Here's one to file under Stranger Than Fiction. When our boys were fifteen months old and I was ready to return to part-time teaching, we found a little nursery school just up the street from my job. Talking to the director, I discovered that our boys would be two of only eight kids, two of whom were another set of identical twin boys, so that the addition of ours made the class 50 percent twin. But that's not the weird part. The weird part began when I visited the classroom and saw that the teacher in charge of the toddlers was the identical twin of the director, and it continued when, a year later, another set of identical twins boys enrolled. Not only would there be four sets of twins on the premises, but all were very identical. Pity the poor singleton kids who had to try to keep track of them all. Our boys, who one might think would be particularly sensitive to the name issue, called two of the twins "Ben-n-Charlie," not unlike the prepubescent islanders addressed "Samneric" (Sam and Eric) in *Lord of the Flies.*

*continued...*

On top of that, they called the director and the teacher by just one name. That, however, wasn't unforgivable, given their names.

When these two women were born, it was near the end of the era of mothers' being surprised in the delivery room when the doctor said, "Wait, that's not all you get!" Indeed, their mother had had no idea. Their parents had picked out one boy name, and if it were a girl, intended to name her Melody. Stymied by the arrival of a second girl, they punted and named her twin Melodia. Seriously. I never even bother to correct my kids when they call each of them "Teacher."

Naming something makes it real. This is the basic premise of all good writing and all effective psychotherapy, and it's true for naming babies, too. Names are opportunities to stress individuality, not collectivity. Let your last name do the group work. Juliet Capulet was wrong when she declared, "That which we call a rose/By any other name would smell as sweet." While it would indeed *actually* smell as sweet, we may *perceive* it differently if it were called Bob. Similarly, each of your children deserves a name that can be perceived by the world as indicative of a single, valued individual. It might be worth bringing an extended list of possibilities to the hospital and waiting to check these kids out first before literally identifying them, too. You may find that your number one choice of names for girls—Kathleen—doesn't fit your dark-eyed, raven-haired baby as well as you had expected, and perhaps you ought to move on to choice number two, Francesca.

We named our boys Grant and Walt, but in spite of all this advice about individuation, we tend to call them both "Put-That-Down-or-You're-in-a-Big-Time-Out-And-I-Mean-It."

# 9

# Thinking Ahead to Day Care and Work Issues

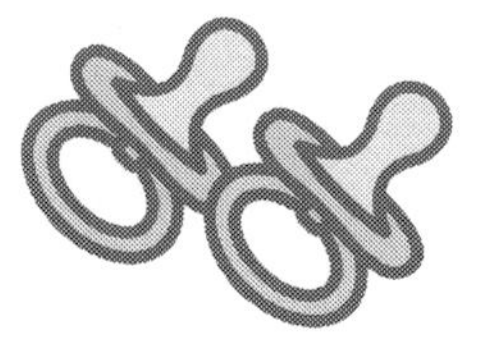

While there may seem to be a sea of women in American suburbs who have left careers in order to raise their children full time, the fact remains that, overall, about 60 percent of women with children under three years old in this country have jobs.[1] You can bet that every one of them has had to do some creative thinking as to how to meet simultaneously the demands of their work and the needs of their children. In any incarnation, the complexity of deciding whether and how to continue to work after children arrive is striking. Going back to work as a new mom is a process fraught with difficult choices.

Having twins can intensify that complexity markedly. Emotionally, you may run into a double dose of the common guilt moms have to wade through when they leave a baby in someone else's arms in order to go to work. You may feel as if you aren't simply finding coverage for an infant but are instead abandoning the project of caring for twins. Or you may feel that it is difficult enough to get to know two babies at once without cutting into the "awake time" you have with them. You may conversely—and even simultaneously—feel an exaggerated need to get back into the world, given the concentration of your babies' demands. It can get knotty. By the same token, having twins may simplify the work decision for you entirely due to the cost of raising two at the same time. In other words, you may have no

---

1. U.S. Department of Labor, U.S. Bureau of Labor Statistics, *Annual Social and Economic Supplements 1975–2006: Current Population Survey*. The percentage of women working who have children 18 years old or under is 70.6%.

choice but to get back to work. Anecdotally, it often seems to be the second or third child who tips the balance and makes it a money-losing situation to work and pay for day care; these could be your second *and* third, and if you return to work, they will both need the same level of expensive day care at the same time.

It is worth thinking about some of these questions before the babies are born, if only to remind yourself not to burn bridges in any direction. While you may be absolutely certain now that you want to quit your job and stay home to raise these babies, it is not totally possible for you to predict how you will feel when they are nine months old during the middle of winter, you haven't left the house for four days, your work friends have stopped checking in on you, and the playgroup you thought would be so fun somehow isn't cutting it for you socially. We rarely talk much about the sometimes inane aspects of spending recurrent full days with little creatures who can't talk and are unapologetically needy. Ask a veteran mom, however, and she will probably admit that there are some truly mind-numbing aspects to this wonderful role. They may be even harder to take if you're used to a challenging, interesting job. While your impending time with the babies seems romantic enough as you sit pregnant and fantasizing in traffic on the way home from another ten hours behind a computer screen, you may be less suited to it than you can imagine, and are perhaps more invested in your work identity than you can know.

On the other hand, if your plan is to return to work after a maternity leave, you may be very surprised by a shift in your perspective that makes that career track seem totally irrelevant and threatening to your new role as mother to these babies. You may find it simply impossible to leave them. You may decide that the challenges of this new role are far more captivating and important to you than those of your former job. You may discover that there's nobody in the world that you could trust to care for your babies as you can, and that you can't compromise on this issue. In any case, it is difficult to know with any precision how you will feel three months, six months, or several years down the road. Whatever flexibility you can instill in your employer's expectations is wise, given this changeability.

Look into the day care situation in your area now, so that you will be prepared later. Obviously, if the plan is to put the babies in day care early, then you need to be pursuing this aggressively. But investigate it regardless of your exact plan and even if your plan is to stay home. At worst, the inquiry will give you a sense of the relative costs of working and staying home. Where I live, it is difficult to find convenient, affordable placement for a young child without having at least a six-month head start. Add to that the fact that you need two slots in the same age grouping, and you can see why this takes forethought. Take tours of local nursery schools, ask moms of older kids where their kids have been while they worked, study the nanny market in your area on the Internet (if you are near a city, http://www.craigslist.org is a hotbed of nanny marketing), and contact Mothers of Twins groups to find out whose twins are graduating out of nanny care into kindergarten, as you may be able to inherit a trained twin nanny.

Like so many elements of raising twins, their exact care arrangement requires some adaptability and is difficult to determine ahead of time. There are human elements involved—largely, yours—that demand an open mind to midstream changes. Yes, you need a plan. But you also need the foresight to know that it can't be written in granite. Or if it is, you should at least use washable markers.

# Part II
# The First Month

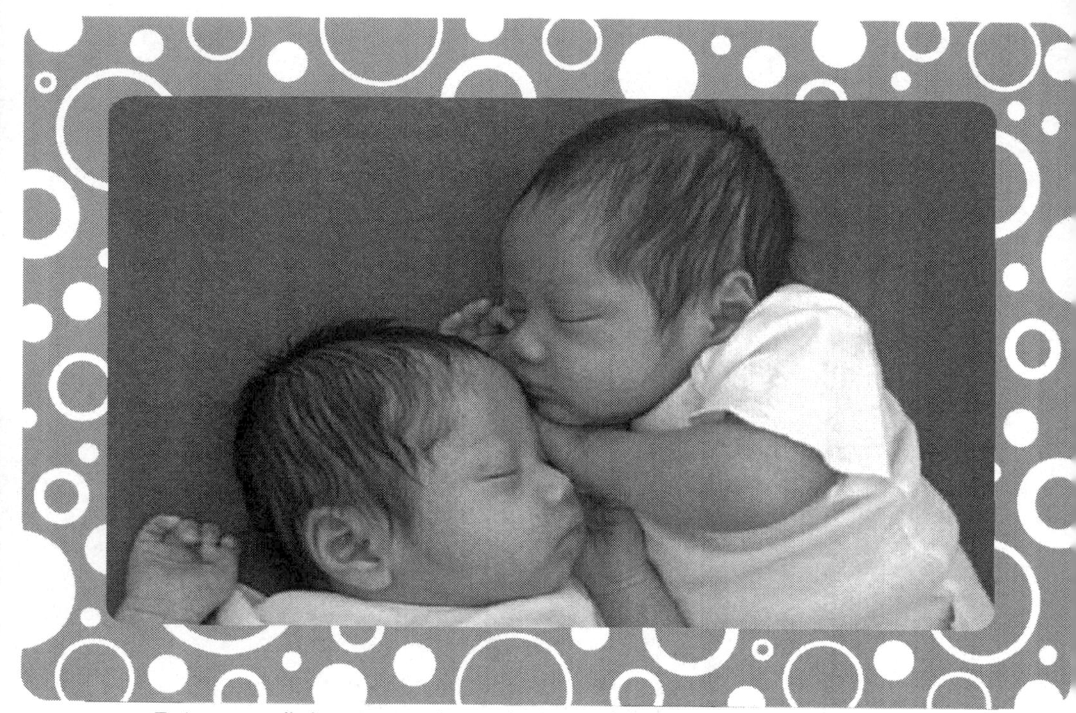

Twins generally love to snuggle together, mimicking their closeness in the womb.

Photo courtesy of Laarni Bulan

New parents are generally exhausted but ecstatic during the first forty-eight hours with their baby, doped up as they are on the adrenaline of miracle (and sometimes some pretty killer psycho-pharmaceuticals for Mom). Braced for the onslaught of neonatal needs that their baby-owning friends have warned them about, they are ready to serve, adore, photograph, pass around, and generally fawn, gloat, and dote over this creature. And in response, for two or three days, the baby does absolutely nothing but sleep incessantly, squinting those groggy little eyes open just long enough to blink a few times, as if to say, "What planet is this?" before passing out again.

It is surely this short-lived period that produced the metaphorical "to sleep like a baby," because it sure ain't the next two years...unless the simile was originally meant to signify sleeping unpredictably, lightly, irritatingly off the schedule of the rest of one's family, and oh yeah, rarely for more than a couple of hours at a time. In short, after a day or two of "sleeping like a baby," babies don't sleep like babies again until college. Meanwhile, however, the new parents have convinced themselves that, "Say! How hard can this be? We've got a great little sleeper here!" Then they take her home and she wakes up, and life as they knew it is utterly finished. If babies weren't designed this way, embedded with this misleading preliminary prank, they would all be left at the hospital. It's just nature's way of making sure we claim all our belongings before leaving the place. As an added little cosmic joke, babies spring to life on the exact day that our birth-miracle adrenaline dries up and Mom's milk comes in, so that both parents are totally spent and one of them is crying incessantly.

Yes, right around day three, babies stop sleeping and start making demands. This will be their approach for the next twenty years or so, but will seem most intense right now. At this point, the circus of caring for your twins is entering the big top and the show is starting, with or without you. Hopefully you will have previously taken my advice and cleared the calendar, the home, and the mind of all other immediate pursuits beyond caring for these babies. But what will it look like, exactly?

# 10

# Life with Two Newborns

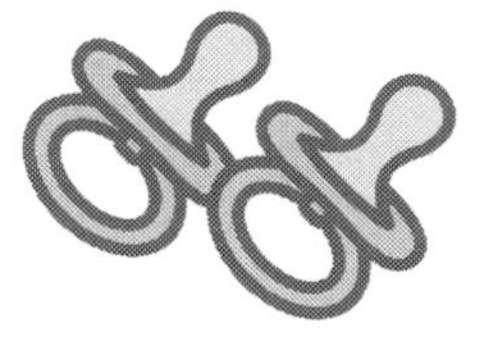

I remember getting home from the hospital with our twins, filling the requisite yardage of film (both video and still) with images of their arrival, putting them down on the floor in their car seats, and thinking, "Now what do we do with them?" For a couple of days, we mostly stared at their slumbering, angelic little mugs. But eventually they roused, hungry as bears emerging from the cave, and the fun began. The best description I have heard for looking after infant twins is that it is like painting the Golden Gate Bridge. That is, the Golden Gate Bridge is so long that by the time the paint crew finishes painting it from end to end, they have to start again back at the beginning with the next coat. Similarly, in the first months of having twins, one cycles repeatedly through the changing, feeding, burping, swaddling, and putting to sleep of each baby, only to begin the process over and over and over again.

Now, some basic research on the history of the Golden Gate Bridge indicates that, unless one factors in the heights, the painters actually have it much easier than do the parents of twins, as it turns out that they in fact only do random touch-ups as needed; the "repeated coats" concept is an urban myth. The image, however, conveys the repetition and relentlessness of babies' requirements in the beginning, and the scaling of heights is similar to the occasional fear you may experience as you wonder if you can actually do this. (You can. Just keep your eyes on what's right in front of you and don't look out at the horizon.)

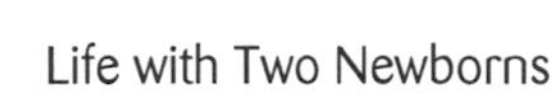

## Coping with the Crying

In the first three months of a baby's life, he or she has total carte blanche. A baby can quite literally do no wrong. He doesn't even know how to misbehave yet. He can't figure out which of your buttons are most easily pushed. He can't be a good baby or a bad baby. He can only be a baby. By definition, young babies are all about eating and sleeping, and the great majority of their crying has to do with one or both of those. In any case, you're not ever allowed to blame the baby. The cry of a baby is designed to rile you to action, and your action must be about comforting the crying child. *You cannot spoil a child under three months,* and you should never worry that picking up and comforting a newborn will form bad habits or teach her to abuse your services. Unfailingly comforting your infants will *not* create a pair of brats; it will create close bonds between you and your babies and will develop their trust and sense of security.

The degree to which you can cope with the babies' crying will determine in part how well you hold it together in the early months. If you are unduly rattled by your babies' cries, the experience of caring for them will be more stressful than it is already likely to be on occasion. Whether you're calm or a mess, it's a good bet that you are going to eventually figure out the best and most efficient way to get the babies' needs met. Your coping or not coping with the crying will mostly affect your own mental health.

### Keep the Faith

You have simply got to cultivate an ability, when two babies are screeching at once and the phone is ringing and the dog is barking, to stand there and laugh for a moment before springing into action. This situation, while nerve-racking, is perfectly normal in a household with two infants. Two factors—your laughter and your faith that this is a period of time that *will end* and give way to calmer months—are the two most crucial tools for getting yourself to those calmer months in one piece.

Because a baby can do no wrong and because she cannot *be* wrong about her needs when she cries (she hasn't learned to fake it yet), you will spend the majority of the first few months with your babies simply answering those needs.

## Is There a Basic Plan?

Recently several books have attempted to help new parents manage and organize their babies' needs into some sort of plan. While I understand the impulse, I do think that any hope of doing so needs to be cautious at best—especially when dealing with two babies at once. A true "schedule" of eating and sleeping doesn't generally emerge during the first month. That said, babies can be quite predictable, and an effort to orchestrate ourselves and our schedules around their predicted needs seems totally right-headed to me. The basic idea presented in these books is that babies can either eat, then sleep, then play…or they can sleep, then eat, then play. ("Play" at this stage means being awake and engaged but not eating.)

Given that these are pretty much the only three things a baby can do at this point, it is not terribly revolutionary to suggest that they do so in some sequence. When the baby is calm, fed, and awake, the mother might be able to seize the moment to claim some sanity-saving time for herself. I'm all for that. Your problem, of course, is that such a proposition would require *two* calm, fed babies, and simple logic will tell you that this scenario is statistically unlikely much of the time. The goal is to make it happen as often as possible, knowing full well that it is a bonus when it does. There are a couple of ways to try.

### Pick a Strategy

Assuming that you have not, in some fit of misguided maternal machis*ma,* attempted to handle the first weeks alone, you will have at least one other parent, grandparent, or sister-type with whom to share baby duties at the beginning. We found that the best labor scenario at this stage was two baby workers and one household worker at any given moment, and we rotated roles pretty regularly. Note that "household" is a very general term that includes the care of older children. At any given moment, the two baby handlers have, as a team, several options as to how to take care of the babies together. The first approach is your basic *We'll Burn That Bridge When We Come To It No-Plan* plan, i.e., playing it by ear. With two people, this can actually work, providing the team is one that communicates well. According to this plan, when a baby cries, you look at each other and quickly decide what to do and who will do it; the team at regular intervals arm wrestles for the right to nap.

A second, more disciplined approach is your basic *Divide and Conquer Plan.* Under this plan, you are each assigned one baby to care for over a set length of time. When your baby cries, you act; when your baby sleeps, you do, too. A third approach is the *Tandem Tag Plan*, by which one member handles two babies solo while the other one sleeps and then they switch. There are advantages to each tactic: the first is the most flexible; the second may be the least stressful; and the third, while demanding that each of you is able to care for both babies alone, rewards you with the biggest chunks of sleep. The important thing to remember for all of these is that we are not talking about a daytime shift or even a double shift; these are round-the-clock shifts. This is why there is an element of sleep involved in each scenario.

It is likely that you will end up cobbling together elements of each plan and fashioning them into your own method of getting the needs of the whole family met. For the first few weeks, you and another caretaker—who may or may not be the same person at all times—will be following some version of these plans in order to make the babies' transition to your home, and into the world, as calming and comforting as possible. Meanwhile, you must yourself get *some* sleep

if you are to be able to keep up this pace. Heroics won't help anyone. Trust your team with the babies and go to sleep whenever you have a chance, be it for five minutes or five hours.

A working goal, besides the obvious one of keeping the kids happy and fed, is to get you to the point of being comfortable staying alone with your babies for extended periods. Only you will know when you are ready for this, and you should bear in mind that it is totally normal *not* to feel ready for it for many weeks. If you were at your physical peak, rather than recovering from a twin birth (not to mention the pregnancy) and dealing with a surplus of hormones, even then the idea of caring for two babies alone would probably give you pause. As you get to know each of your babies in these first weeks, however, your confidence will mushroom. Every time you move a baby from a state of agitation to state of tranquility, you will see that you can do this. You will have the tools, and with practice, you will become very good at this.

Depending on when you are ready to handle the babies alone, it is possible that they will be approaching an age at which they can stick to the program a bit. If you are taking care of the babies with someone, you will have the opportunity to try to keep the babies pretty much on a schedule of eating at the same time and sleeping at the same time. This isn't as likely a scenario once you are alone. While it *is* possible and is a total time-saver to feed them at the same time, either by breast or by bottle, the resettling and putting to sleep of a baby often requires some focused one-on-one attention, and only an octopus mother could truly handle two at once in this way.

A more reasonable goal would be to keep them in close consecutive order, so that you feed Baby A, let her hang out sated and happily close to you as you feed Baby B, let Baby B then hang out as you put Baby A to bed, and then put Baby B to bed. (Repeat cycle for a number of months...) Once you are able to feed them at the same time, the only real split will happen as you are settling one to sleep

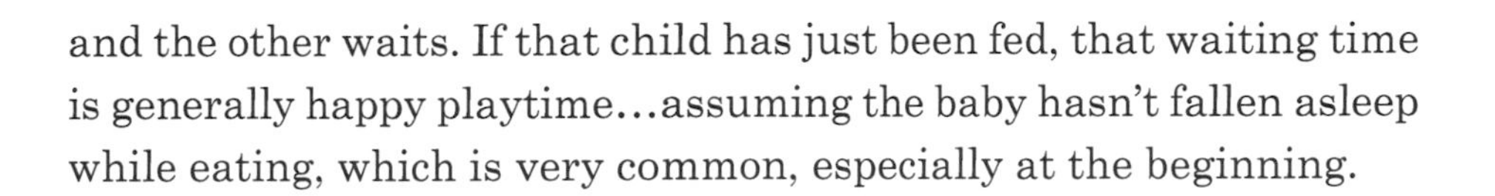

and the other waits. If that child has just been fed, that waiting time is generally happy playtime...assuming the baby hasn't fallen asleep while eating, which is very common, especially at the beginning.

## Patterns, Not Promises

There are advantages to both the sleep-eat-play order and, conversely, the eat-sleep-play order. The main advantage for a twin mom in having them eat immediately as they wake up is that the awake time is calmer, given that they are just-fed and happy. The tricky part is that they awaken quite hungry and may both want to be fed at once (if they awaken at the same time), and this can be quite stressful if you're not able to feed both right away. The main advantage of having them eat, then sleep, then play is that the plan accounts for their tendency to get knocked out cold by a good feeding and doesn't necessitate long periods of getting them to sleep. Again, though, before you start writing either plan in a Sharpie on the family calendar, remember that these are patterns, not promises.

Every day, at some point (or perhaps many), you are going to have to wing it. Sometimes it will be for dreadful reasons, such as because neither of them slept for more than fifteen minutes at a time during the night and both needed more formula than they've ever taken just to be somewhat consoled. Or it may be for wonderful reasons, such as you were planning to feed them both around 6, but your daughter slept until 6:30, giving you some precious alone time with your son. There will be an enormous amount of improvisation on a daily basis, but if you have a basic structure in mind, you are likely to feel a bit more control. Just don't be too disappointed if somehow the babies don't get the memo about the day's projected schedule. In very short order you will become more adaptable than you knew you could be.

It does take some practice, however. In particular, what takes practice is not just calming the babies, but calming yourself. Over

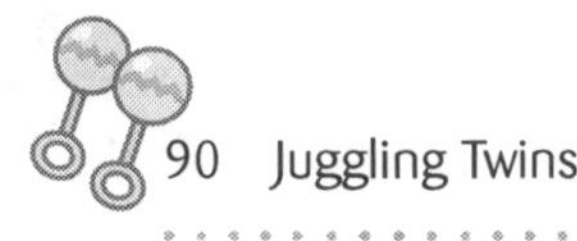


the first few weeks, you need to learn to (1) breathe deeply when a baby (or two) cries, (2) assess their needs, and then (3) provide for them patiently. Your reaction may not immediately restore order to a flailing, unsettled baby, or to the scene of two of them unraveling, but eventually it *will,* if you can remain calm and deliberately use the comforting methods that you know to work with your children. While feeding, burping, changing, swaddling, swaying, shushing, rocking, and otherwise pacifying babies are all important skills, the truly crucial ability that you are trying to perfect is your capacity for remaining unruffled, steady, and composed. This poised self-control will not necessarily be your instinctual response—yours may be something closer to horror, total exasperation, flight, or a piercing primal scream—but it is important on so many levels, beyond the obvious help it is to an upset child to be cared for by a steady, self-possessed parent.

Try to see your children's needs as natural, understandable, and solvable, and learn to address them methodically. Over the long haul, this will serve not only your babies, but also your own mental health. Bracing yourself for the onslaught of more crying may be a natural defense mechanism, but in the end, it's one that takes an emotional and physical toll on you and prescribes your babies the role of the enemy. The healthier approach takes practice, but it is worth your conscious effort, for their sakes and yours, to see this intense period of time together as a venture you are all embarking on as a team. Some days, this will be easier than others. Some days, it will be impossible. On those truly tough days, when my babies seemed utterly inconsolable and I would have sold my soul for just one hour of sleep, I sometimes remembered Macbeth's remark that, "Come what come may/Time and the hour runs through the roughest day."[1] Of course, things didn't end so well for Macbeth, so perhaps

1. William Shakespeare, *Macbeth,* act I, sc. III,11. 145–6.

he's not the best mentor for patience. The bottom line is that you need the confidence to realize that your head will still be attached to your neck at the end of this play, and the more composed you can be during your performance, the better off everyone will be.

# 11

# The Daily Chart

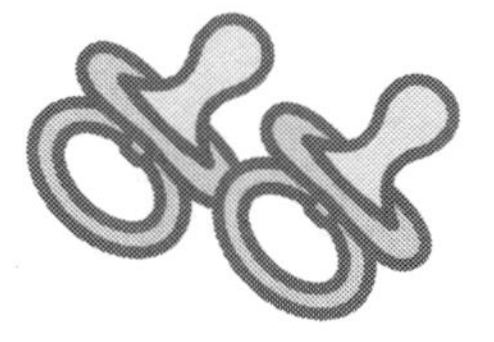

The key to maintaining any semblance of sanity in the first few months with your babies is a very simple tool: a daily chart. This is true regardless of whether you feed your babies formula or breastfeed them. Charting what, when, and how much your babies eat and expel is crucial for several reasons.

Under normal circumstances, you would not be able to remember or keep straight when two different babies have eaten, or how much… and let's face it, these will *not* be normal circumstances, where your brain function is concerned. Let me put this as kindly as possible: you won't be running on all your cerebral cylinders when your babies are newborns. No matter how focused you are during a feeding, a half hour later, you will not be able to recall whom you have fed or how much. All you will remember is sitting on a sofa with someone small who was sucking away. Even if your twins aren't identical, you will be hard-pressed to name that baby; they are both small and look similar enough when seen from above through sleepy eyes. Feeding two infants every couple of hours can amount to as many as twenty sessions a day. Eventually, these feedings will all run together in your mind, and you'll be damned if you can come up with the amount eaten or the name of the baby who ate it. At that point, you may in fact be damned if you can remember your own name. And whereas your own name is immaterial now, you really do need to know how much is going in and out of each kid.

Even if you could miraculously recall every ounce, every moment, and every nuance of every feeding, writing it all down would still

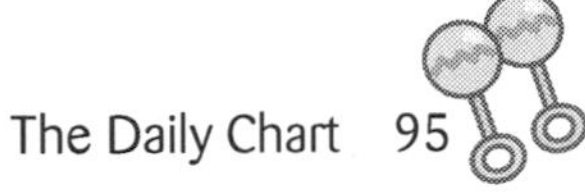

be desirable in order to make the transfer of that information to other caretakers seamless. You won't be—you can't be—the boss of the world for every shift. When your deputies take over, you want them to have all the information they need right at the ready. Don't require them to elicit it from you in your addled, possibly semi-conscious state. Let them simply flip through the charts. Similarly, when you are ready to resume your reign, you can just review the shift report to see what has transpired while you were sleeping and dreaming of simpler days (...you know that dream...the one where you, slim you, are on a beach somewhere with a novel...).

Start the chart the first day you come home from the hospital. After a few days of keeping it, you will be able to see important patterns and important absences of patterns. It was the very earliest of charts, for example, that helped us realize that our boys were not getting enough breast milk, as it became clear that their bowel movements had become much less frequent after the second week than they had been during the first. While their weight loss wasn't as apparent to us—we barely even knew them yet and couldn't really perceive it visually—their extended periods without pooping were hints that we needed to call the pediatrician. I couldn't have known without those clues that I wasn't producing enough breast milk for both of them. Without the charts, I might have simply figured that some other diaper changer was getting nailed with the poopy ones. That discovery led to our getting a breastfeeding consultant who helped me enormously, and in short order, the kids resumed gaining weight. Keeping charts helps to solve all sorts of medical and behavioral puzzles. It also begins the very important work of differentiating the babies.

For example, while you may not perceive how frequent it is that one baby eats just two ounces while the other manages three, seeing it written twenty times over a few days will show you an emerging pattern that could be useful to you or to your babies' pediatrician. It

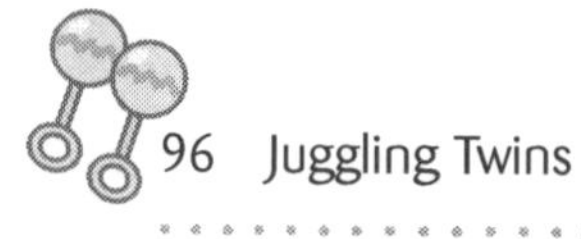



is your primary tool for trying to answer the many questions you will have when the children are newborns. If the baby who is starting to seem colicky is only eating half as much as the more settled baby, perhaps she's actually hungry but is struggling with gas, or is routinely falling asleep at the breast before she has finished eating. Having the information charted lets you put together a reasoned response to behaviors without working simply from memory.

Though our twins were on an orderly feeding schedule at about three months, we continued to keep the charts until they were over six months old. In the first three months, our documentation was focused on food, but during months three to six, the charts became a great tool for getting their napping and sleeping schedule sorted out. For those who believe in some degree of sleep training, it can be especially helpful to have a record of when naps happened, how they were initiated, if (and how long) a baby cried before putting himself to sleep, and how long he eventually slept. As we watched our boys progress in their ability to get themselves to sleep, the chart reassured us that we were on the right track and should continue to gut out the hard work of teaching them to put themselves to sleep. It shouldn't be surprising, either, that we could easily see patterned relationships between hours of sleep each child attained and his or her ability to cope with life the next day. If you're not already a convert, the chart can make you a believer in the religion of early bedtimes and sacred nap routines. (We have our own sect and are fairly fanatical.)

There are other benefits to using a chart, too. It can be fun later to flip back to the week before a growth spurt and see how the whole thing was in the cards, as one or both of the babies were sucking in the calories to get ready for the explosion.

As the notebook swells with days of recorded caretaking, it starts to take on the character of a baby journal, often with margin notes that will later recall for you both the incredible attention to detail that became so routine and also your emerging understanding of each child.

You will some day marvel at your serious narratives about gassiness and will be reminded, nostalgically perhaps, about how the presence or absence of this gas was *a really big deal for you* at this stage, affecting the whole family's quality of life. When your kids are six years old, it will bring a tear to your eye to see the exclamation points you scribbled on the chart the day the first smile came.

Our thick notebook of daily charts lives with all our twins' other baby memorabilia and occasionally gets flipped through for its ability to return us instantly to the intensity of those first months, when life was entirely devoted to the full-throttle, relentless needs of our little guys. Because of that intensity, moreover, we had little opportunity or energy to maintain the sweet baby journals our friends gave us, but our notebook tells the story perfectly, complete with occasional coffee stains, some indecipherable messages written with the wrong hand because the writing hand was full of baby, and sweet, supportive notes from caretakers we haven't seen since the babies were still babies. Reading it over now and then makes us proud of having gotten through those months in one piece, with two healthy children in tow.

## Sample Daily Chart

Below is a sample chart. Ideally, several months' worth of charts would be printed, hole-punched at the top, and popped into a three-ring binder that can be flipped up easily.

DAILY CHART

DATE: ________________

Name ________________

Name ________________

| Time | Minutes | Amt. | B/F | L/R | Wet | BM | Notes | | Time | Minutes | Amt. | B/F | L/R | Wet | BM | Notes |
|---|---|---|---|---|---|---|---|---|---|---|---|---|---|---|---|---|
| 1 | | | | | | | | | 1 | | | | | | | |
| 2 | | | | | | | | | 2 | | | | | | | |
| 3 | | | | | | | | | 3 | | | | | | | |
| 4 | | | | | | | | | 4 | | | | | | | |
| 5 | | | | | | | | | 5 | | | | | | | |
| 6 | | | | | | | | | 6 | | | | | | | |
| 7 | | | | | | | | | 7 | | | | | | | |
| 8 | | | | | | | | | 8 | | | | | | | |
| 9 | | | | | | | | | 9 | | | | | | | |
| 10 | | | | | | | | | 10 | | | | | | | |
| 11 | | | | | | | | | 11 | | | | | | | |
| 12 | | | | | | | | | 12 | | | | | | | |
| | | | | | | | | | | | | | | | | |

REMARKS:

- Start each day at midnight, so that feeding #1 for each baby is the first one that happens after midnight.
- Use one side of the chart for each twin and keep those sides for the duration. Write the names every time, so that you are sure in a glance of whose day you're reporting.
- *As soon as a feeding ends,* go right to the book and report it. Do not trust yourself to do this after you have done a few dishes or made a phone call. Not only will you draw a complete blank as to the exact details of the feeding, but there's a pretty good chance you'll forget to write it at all. Make it your routine to finish a feeding, change and settle the baby, and then report in. Keep the notebook in a central location, like on a kitchen counter or dining room table, where it is easily accessible, won't get covered with newspapers, mail, or dinner, and can live for months unmolested.
- Under the appropriate child's name, write the time that you *began* the feeding. In the next column, write the number of minutes it took for the baby to finish the feeding. If you are using a bottle, either for formula or pumped milk, write the number of ounces the baby drank. Specify in the next column whether the ounces were expressed breast milk or formula. If it was a combination of both, you might write, for example, 2/1, meaning two ounces of breast milk and one of formula. If you are using formula exclusively, this and the next column are irrelevant. If you breastfed the baby, skip the "amount" column, but write in the next column either L (for left) or R (for right) to indicate which breast the baby suckled. In the last columns, put a check if the baby was either wet or had a bowel movement when you changed him. Finally, in the "notes" column, you might indicate if the baby was especially fussy, if she fell asleep while eating, if there was anything particularly colorful or riveting about her poop, if the entire feeding was subsequently hurled down your back, etc.

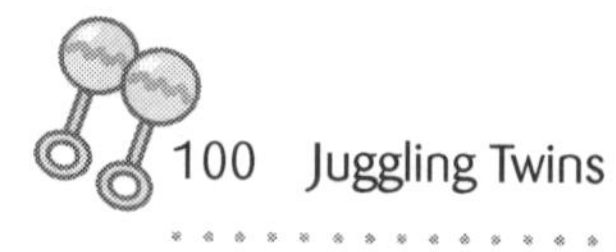


- At the bottom, under "remarks," write notes to incoming help ("Let me know if there's more spitting up," "May not take much at next feeding, did a great job," or "Is it me, or does she look like Truman Capote?"), report milestones ("Yay! He slept for five hours straight!"), or give general updates ("Three straight hours of crying today! And then the babies started crying, too!").

# 12

# Feeding Two Newborns

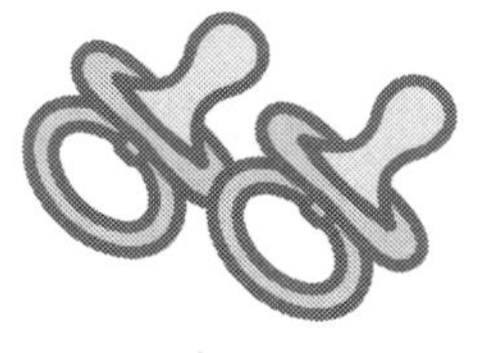

In the beginning, parents of a newborn feel as if their child eats pretty much nonstop. And how does one begin to measure nonstop times two? Well, you can look at the basic reality that it can take a very young baby more than a half an hour to consume a feeding. If she does this twelve times in 24 hours, that's at least six hours a day. Simple math then tells you that, with twins, you will be feeding your babies, collectively, over twelve hours per day. That's if the babies only eat every two hours; some eat on the hour at the beginning, particularly if they are on the small side or if they are breastfeeding.

Suffice it to say that feeding your babies is going to be your primary occupation and preoccupation for a while: it will be the way in which you spend most of your waking hours and the subject about which you may devote a substantial amount of mental energy. If this sounds dreadful, like a sentence to sit for months while the world turns without you, then you're forgetting something important. Feeding one's infant can be one of the most satisfying, mystically gorgeous experiences a parent has, be it mother or father, breast or bottle. Those many hours may now seem onerous in their number, but if you recognize in advance that everything else will be on hold for a while, and if you give yourself permission to *put all else on hold for your babies' sakes,* then you will enable yourself to see all those feeding sessions as chances to regroup and relax, connect with each infant, and experience the intense emotional fulfillment of bringing comfort and contentment to your babies.

## Nursing vs. Bottle-Feeding Formula

Every mother must decide whether she will be nursing her baby or bottle-feeding formula. The benefits your baby attains through breastfeeding are clear and have been the subject of a steady stream of attention in the mass media, as a trickle down from the attention the subject has received in the medical world. There is no doubt that breast milk, formulated perfectly for a baby's needs and adaptive to the developmental changes in those needs, is the food of choice for babies. For the mother of twins, the list of the benefits of breastfeeding is even longer:

### Benefits of Breastfeeding

- It can provide intimate bonding time with each baby when they are nursed separately, allowing the mother to get to know each child apart from the other. It also offers each baby a form of individual comfort that will be available until he or she is weaned.
- It is absolutely beneficial in the case of premature babies, who need every nutritional advantage they can get. The milk of a mother of premature babies has more protein and amino acids than it will at the actual due date, in anticipation of the babies' increased need for quick weight gain and concentrated nutrition. (Amazing, isn't it?)
- Formula is very expensive, and you will go through cases of it if you use it exclusively.
- Because the hassles of bottle preparation and cleanup are doubled with twins, breastfeeding can be much more efficient and convenient—particularly in the middle of the night.

Many sources of advice to twin moms suggest that breastfeeding is the obvious way to go, and that it is a cinch because we have two breasts and the body is the perfect baby-feeding machine, capable of adjusting quickly to the task of providing for two. Breastfeeding is a

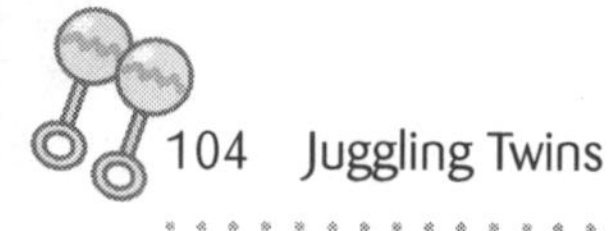


model of perfect supply and demand, they assure us. I was certainly encouraged by these buoyant promises when I was planning to breastfeed my twins and was so happy about the prospect of repeating the glorious nursing experience I had had with my older daughter. I know of many, many women for whom these promises came true, and breastfeeding their twins was a wonderful, gratifying experience for them and their babies. I think it's worth honestly noting, at the same time, that while our bodies may in fact have the capacity to adjust to the nutritional demands of two, it is not always a perfect adjustment, and breastfeeding two babies can be very challenging on a number of levels. To portray it as the perfectly natural, obvious choice can be a setup for frustration and disappointment. Not every mother of twins will find it plausible to stick with breastfeeding. There are plenty of moms of twins who know from the start that they can't commit to the effort, and their decision to formula-feed from the beginning is in that case the right one entirely. Baby formula is a truly viable and healthy solution when breastfeeding is not workable.

Just as there are excellent reasons to breastfeed twins, there are also compelling reasons to bottle-feed formula:

## Benefits of Formula Feeding

- Breast milk digests more quickly, which means even more feedings. While this might not be a reasonable factor in deciding how to feed a singleton, the prospect of feeding two babies every ninety minutes or so might not seem practicable to you.
- While it may be considered a perfect system of supply and demand, not all moms are in fact able to generate a perfect supply for two. This is perhaps even more likely in an older mom, and many of us having twins are older moms. Low supply may mean lots of pumping in an effort to make enough for both, and this may or may not solve the problem.
- Some of the convenience factor of breastfeeding is compromised a bit by having two babies to feed. While you may have felt comfortable nursing

your first baby on a bench at the park or in a corner of your favorite café, for example, nursing two at once is pretty tough to do discreetly and usually involves more attention and exposure. (Usually of your belly. How eager are you to show *that* to the world these days?)

- Some nursing moms of twins describe breastfeeding not in terms of a hallowed, precious time with their babies but more like channeling their inner dairy cow. They simply found the constant nursing to be overwhelming on a number of levels.

## Reality Check

In the interest of full disclosure, I will say here that I hope you decide to try to breastfeed your babies, for the reasons first listed above. But I also hope that you don't make the mistake of convincing yourself that anything short of a perfect, complete, yearlong, nursing-for-two scenario is a failure. As with your entire life ahead of you with twins, you will need to be flexible as you decide and recalculate—perhaps many times—the best feeding arrangement for your brood. You may even be surprised to discover that it works best for everyone if you breastfeed one and bottle-feed the other. That scenario was suggested to me when one of our boys was really struggling to get enough while breastfeeding, and I protested fervently that it would create an unmatchable bond for the nursing child and that the bottle-fed boy would be emotionally disadvantaged, relatively. Our trusted twin expert told me this was nonsense and that bonding is much more complex than suckling. In retrospect, I wish I had listened to her, as pushing through doggedly with both sons was remarkably stressful, not just for me, but sometimes for them as well.

Overall, their experience may have been better had I been willing to let go of the promises of those books that had made me certain my body could do this if only it were signaled that more supply was needed. I stuck with it for eight months, but now wonder if I should have raised the white flag earlier. Obviously, only you can know what

*continued...*

works for you and your babies at any given time. I am always amazed by and congratulatory of women who manage to breastfeed their two babies exclusively for many months. The best plan for any family with twins, however, is the one that allows for the possibility of *any* plan and is able to adjust as you learn to understand their needs... and yours.

## Breastfeeding Two

If you do intend to breastfeed, you will need to continue to consume more calories than prior to your pregnancy. As promising as that sounds, it is likely that your consumption fantasies have never centered on spinach, lean meats, and live-cultured yogurts. Breastfeeding in general requires a conscious effort to eat well and plentifully. Providing for two doesn't require double the calories, but it does require double the consciousness of nutrition's importance in your mission to have milk for two.

The whole process of making milk is truly remarkable, not simply because it results in the perfect food for your children at any given moment, but because your body makes milk not by gathering its components (calcium, iron, protein, etc.) from your diet and transferring them to your breast milk, but instead by making your milk from scratch, as it were. Most women in the world who nurse babies do so while eating less-than-balanced meals; many are in fact nutritionally impoverished. And yet, their bodies can make milk. Good nutrition doesn't affect the quality or composition of your milk; it can, however, affect your ability to make it in the quantity your babies need without exhausting you in the process.[1]

---

1. "Research shows that the mother's diet, her fluid intake, and other factors have little influence on milk production. If the 'milk removal' piece of the puzzle is in place, mothers make plenty of good milk regardless of dietary practices." Linda J. Smith, "How Mother's Milk Is Made," *Leaven* 37, no. 3 (June–July 2001): 54–5, Le Leche League "Resources," http://www.llli.org, (accessed February 29, 2008).

The goal is to feed your body quality nutrition that fuels your production of milk and also helps you cope with the challenges of these first weeks and months. That said, on the days that you fall short of this goal and take-out spare ribs and potato salad are presented to you as dinner, you should feel no guilt as you wipe the barbecue sauce from your chin. Your body will compensate and the babies' nutrition will not be compromised in the ways yours has been that day. The next day, however, you should be back on the nutrition wagon, seeking out copious amounts of foods that act more as fuel than as entertainment or comfort.

The edict to drink more water is already well established for all nursing moms. Again, however, you don't need double the amount of water you would for one. You simply need to be doubly mindful of the need to drink enough. When I left the hospital, one of the party favors they sent home with me was a 4,000-ounce tumbler with a giant flexible straw sprouting out the top. "Drink up!" the nurses said, and I nearly drowned myself trying to please them. If you're paying attention and drinking enough to keep yourself from getting thirsty, you're probably fine.

If this is your first time breastfeeding a baby, be sure to elicit and assimilate all the help and advice you can find from lactation consultants, midwives, and hospital nurses who are present after the babies are born. While it is true that breastfeeding is a natural process, it is not true that we all know deep in our cells exactly how to get a newborn to latch on correctly or how to cope with engorged breasts or nipple pain. Beyond the basics of breastfeeding a baby, moreover, a nursing mother of twins needs to learn how to coordinate her feeding of two. This happens on two levels. The first is figuring out when to feed each one. The second is the more literal coordination, when they are eating together, of arranging two little bodies at your breasts. This trick takes some practice, but there are some tried and true methods.

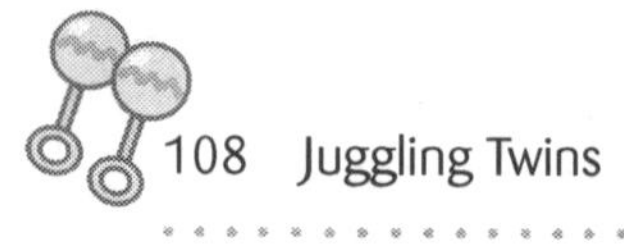


## Tandem Feedings

You should definitely attempt to feed the babies in tandem (one at each breast) at some point when you have the onsite support of a nurse or lactation consultant to help you. For the first days and weeks, though, you will probably be feeding the babies separately, one after the other. Breastfeeding them individually simply makes sense at the beginning. It allows you to work with each baby to establish latching and suckling techniques, and it gives you special time to get to know each baby separately. Because there will be help at the beginning, you shouldn't feel any pressure to "get through" feedings in a timely manner. At some point, however, you will want to try feeding them at the same time, to see what that is like for you and for them. Eventually, there will be some real advantages to having the option of feeding the babies together, as it cuts (nearly) in half the time it takes to feed them. It's a good idea to practice feeding them simultaneously at least once a day.

### Help!

The classic madonna and child scene is modified a bit when there are two children in the picture. Not only does it take some practice to figure out how to position two babies at your breasts in the beginning, but it also takes some assistance. In the first weeks of your attempting to feed them together, you will absolutely need someone to help you throughout the session.

If you are hoping to nurse the babies long-term, you will want to purchase a double nursing pillow designed for twins. This is a rather stiff, covered foam pillow that sits on your lap, wraps around your middle, and has a surface area large enough to hold two babies. Its height brings the babies comfortably to breast level. If you're not sure that you want to invest in this somewhat pricey item, you can get a similar effect by taking about six pillows and mushing them around you from the back of the sofa all the way around to your lap, creating a semisolid shelf for the babies to lie on. By the way, you can't nurse twins in a chair because you won't all fit. Sofas are safest, though it also may be comfortable to nurse in bed. The exact positioning of pillows depends on your shape, the babies' latching, and where you prefer to nurse. Experiment with different arrangements as much as you can while you have help.

In any case, you do need some sort of pillow support for the babies, as you can't independently hold two babies whose necks are still floppy for over half an hour at your breast without breaking your back and possibly making your own neck floppy. You may also want to prop pillows behind you before you even sit down, particularly if you nurse in bed. This is especially helpful when the babies are bigger and are able to kick harder, because it prevents them from attempting kick turns off the back of your seat or your headboard (a good practice to prevent, as they will take your nipple with them on their push-off to the next lap).

Once you have your pillows arranged, have your helper pass you a baby. If there is a visible difference in the degree to which the kids have taken to suckling, put the stronger nurser on first. Once she is happily feeding, have your helper hand you the next baby and then hold the already-nursing baby in place as you settle the next one on your other breast. When the babies are quite small, it's generally easy enough to have them spooning back to belly, each lying in the same direction and each with access to a breast. As they get older and the inside baby no longer has enough room, the positioning generally is the "football hold" or some variation on it, such as one baby in the cradle position and the other in the football hold.

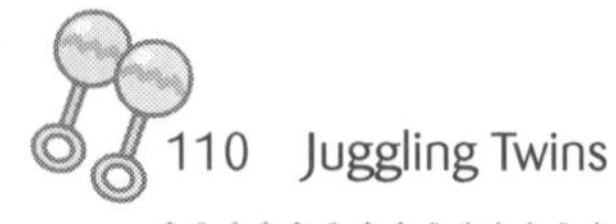



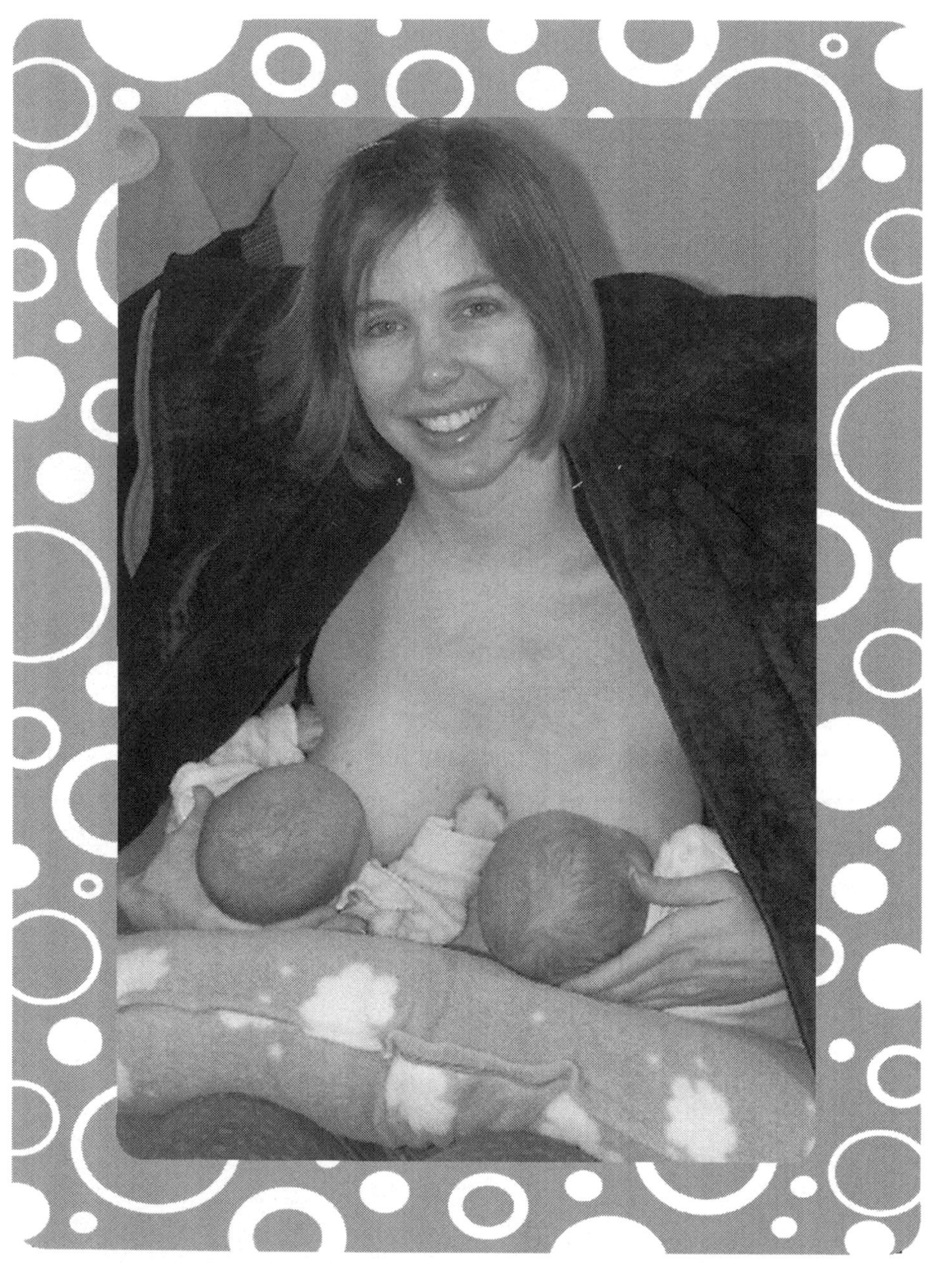

The double football hold. Have someone help you the first time you attempt to get your twins situated simultaneously.

Photo courtesy of Holly Fischer-Engel

With the help of the pillows, you should have your hands free to help the babies, hold their heads closer, readjust their latch, and pick each of them up to burp, individually and gingerly, over your shoulder. Again, all of this takes practice, and your helper should be there every step of the way the first few times, not just as you start to feed them. Have her keep a hand on the back of the nursing baby when you pick her sibling up to get a burp, just to be sure there's nobody rolling off the pillow and onto the floor. Once a baby is finished or nodding off, your helper can take her away while you wrap things up with the other. If you were feeding a single baby who fell asleep, you could safely stand up with him in your arms. Maneuvering two sleeping infants is trickier, and you need to make sure the babies are safe before getting up. Again, it is crucial to have another pair of hands at the start, and you may want to wait until each baby has had a few days to establish breastfeeding before even trying to nurse them together. In any case, you don't want to attempt it alone.

One method that works well is to have one or two C-shaped, stuffed pillow rings made for single babies (often called *Boppies*), in addition to your double nursing pillow. If you place one next to you on the sofa with the opening facing either you or the back of the sofa, you can use it as a safe depository for a sleeping child while you nurse her sibling. Popping her in its center will keep her from rolling off the sofa. A couple of months later, you can also use it to turn a baby on her belly in order to burp her while nursing the other, or to have her hang out happily with a toy while you tend to her twin.

About half of the women I know who nursed twins regularly did so in tandem fashion. The other half ended up feeding one after the other. I generally fell into this latter group, as deeply as the efficiency of feeding them together appealed to me. The coordination aspect wasn't the challenge for me, ultimately, though it certainly was at the beginning. I simply found the actual nursing from two

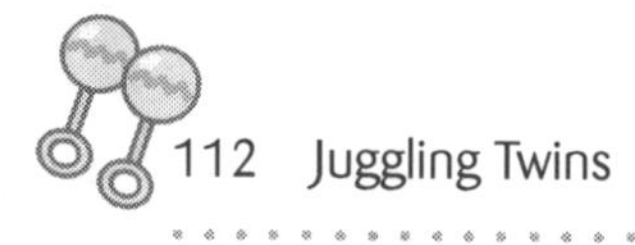


breasts to be overstimulating and overwhelming. Whereas nursing one baby felt to me like gently floating down a tranquil river, nursing two was more like swimming in Class V rapids; it was just too much. I know other moms who felt similarly, but also know plenty who had no such feeling and loved feeding their twins together. Some feel it created more closeness in the children, too, as they snuggled in together repeatedly every day.

Regardless of your outcome, it will undoubtedly be the case that breastfeeding will become easier as your babies gain neck control and become proficient nursers who can clear out a breast in less than half the time they took as newborns. By the time most babies are in the second half of their first year, they are able to take in a full feeding in about ten minutes and rarely need help burping. These changes alone make issues of coordination easier to deal with. Many women don't regularly feed both at one time for a number of weeks but then do so exclusively once all three members of the team have perfected their techniques. By a year, many women report being able to flop down on a sofa without any pillows as the kids position themselves and cozy on in, needing little help at all.

## Separate Feedings

If you do feed them one after the other, you will want to become attuned to signs of their impending hunger, so that you can feed one peacefully without having the other unravel entirely while waiting her turn. This is a good skill to learn in general (you should practice it with yourself too, rather than eating ten minutes after you get hungry), but it is especially important when one baby will be waiting for his turn to eat. It is stressful for all three—perhaps you more than the others—to try to conduct a feeding while one ravenous baby roars right next to a suckling sibling. Learn to recognize the signs of hunger that precede crying: mouth activity such as opening, rooting, or lip-licking or -smacking; hand-to-mouth activity, especially sucking on fingers; movement of the head back and forth; and nuzzling against your chest.

If you feed the babies as they are approaching hunger rather than entering it, you should be able to entertain the waiting baby in his boppy pillow with toys, a pacifier, or a finger for him to suck on. It was this scenario, actually, that converted us from reluctant pacifier-parents to absolute believers in the power of the Almighty Binkie. A pacifier could do just that—*pacify* the waiting baby better and longer than we could as he waited to eat. We eliminated them early, at three months, which took approximately one minute to do. That is, we threw them out. Done deal. Meanwhile, they had absolutely saved us during those first twelve weeks, not only for the baby-in-queue scenario, but also for lulling them into sleep or settling them when they were simply out of sorts. When we see toddlers with binkies, however, we are always glad that we initiated the withdrawal program well before there was any true addiction.

There is always the possibility, as happened regularly with me, that your babies will still be hungry after having seemingly cleared you out of milk. When this happens, you always have the option of supplementing feedings with formula in bottles. While some experts worry that doing so will cause "nipple confusion" and induce the baby to choose bottles over mom, this was not the case for us, and our twin nanny mentor assured us that if it is learned early enough, babies can go back and forth between the two effortlessly. Ours did. Obviously, if they are able to do so without compromising the breastfeeding program, they are then able to take bottles of your expressed milk from others, which creates the potential for mom to have breaks from the constant feedings. The mothers of babies who are able both to nurse and take bottles may look forward to full nights of sleep at some point, or a dinner out in an outfit that doesn't have flaps that unsnap at her breasts. Still, many mothers resist the introduction of artificial nipples altogether, having worked hard to establish effective breastfeeding. Complementing a nursing session with a bottle may also inadvertently start you on a slippery slope of supply issues if you don't then pump in order to simulate the demand that is now being met with an "outside" bottle. This is an especially important consideration in the first six to eight weeks, as you are building your supply and establishing habits.

## Other Considerations

Never sit down to begin a feeding without being prepared to be there for a long time. While your instinct when you hear your children cry will be to get food into their squalling maws as fast as is humanly possible, you will need to train your body to react instead by rushing to the bathroom. That's right. When your babies are hungry, immediately go pee, because you are not going to want to stop a perfect feeding or remove a sleeping child from your shoulder in a half hour when your bladder kicks in. After you have done this and have washed your hands well, you should place next to where you will sit a preloaded basket or bucket or bag of everything you could possibly need, including burp cloths, pacifiers, baby toys, bottles, water, a snack, something to read, pen and paper, and the phone. If you have one particular place where you will always nurse, you can leave your supplies there and have them at the ready, so that you need only grab a drink before starting.

Two other nursing reminders: Changing a baby before she is fed is a good way to wake her up for the meal and is preferable to changing her after eating, as it is best for her that you don't lay her flat for over a half hour after she has eaten. Secondly, you may choose to feed each baby from his or her "own" breast, or you may switch them up every time in order to ensure a more even supply.

## Pumping

Pumping your breasts for milk with a high-quality electric machine (don't skimp; the weenie ones are slooow, and you don't have the time to spare) may be something you want to consider doing for either of two basic reasons. The first is if you plan to leave your babies at any point while they are still nursing, be it for a night out or a return to full-time work. The other is if you are trying to increase your supply of milk. If you are hoping to feed your babies exclusively with your milk but can't be with them for every hour of every day, then you will need to stockpile some of it in the freezer for other caretakers to use in feeding them in your absence. If you are going to be returning to work, you may need to pump not simply to fill the freezer but also to maintain your supply. Pumping is second-rate to baby mouths as an extractor or creator of breast milk, but many women find that adding it to the routine does in fact help to maintain supply, both in your body and in the freezer.

By and large, women pump for all sorts of reasons and on all sorts of schedules. Some stockpile milk that they pump in the morning, when their supply is at its peak, to give to their babies toward the end of the day when they are exhausted, their supply is depleted, and the babies are fussy. Some simply stash the stuff for unspecified bottle-feeding later, knowing that it is absolutely liquid gold. Others pump exclusively and bottle-feed their breast milk because one or both of their babies has trouble nursing. Some pump one breast while feeding with the other (much easier with a singleton, clearly). Others feed one baby, then the other, and then pump. In any configuration, it is another aspect of breastfeeding that requires a serious dedication of time and energy, which is another reason to rent or buy a good-quality pump rather than an underpowered, battery-operated imposter.

The most obvious benefit of successful pumping is that it allows others to feed the babies on occasion without having to use formula.

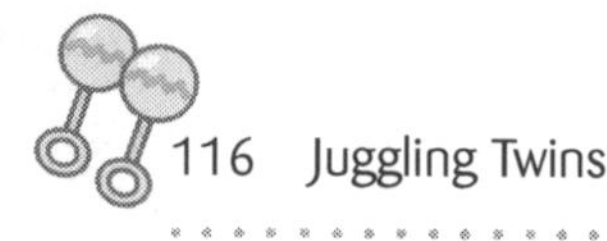


While pumping requires even more time at the point in your life when you have none to spare, seeing bags of breast milk lined up in the freezer brings its own satisfaction. We learned to lay the bags level to freeze, so that we could then "file" the flat frozen packages by date and use the oldest one first. (In order to do this, be sure to find the breast milk storage bags that have zip-tops; the twisty-tie versions can't do this.)

> Though it's not an image I care to recall any more than is absolutely necessary, I became quite adept at pumping both breasts at once. I even learned to check e-mail simultaneously. This made me feel a bit more human: it separated me from the rest of the herd, in that cows are notoriously clumsy with computers.

## Bottle-Feeding

### General Guideline for Feeding Infants[2]

2 ½ times baby's weight = number of ounces per day

For example:

6 lb. baby needs 15 oz. per day

8 lb. baby needs 20 oz. per day

Whether you are using bottles either by plan, by default, for "comps" (supplementary, or complementary, bottles), or for occasional

2 Jan Riordan, *Breastfeeding and Human Lactation,* 3rd ed. (Jones & Bartlett Publishers, Inc., 2004), 194.

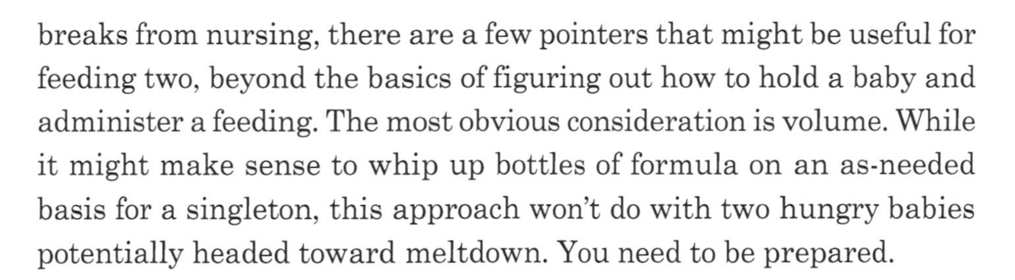

breaks from nursing, there are a few pointers that might be useful for feeding two, beyond the basics of figuring out how to hold a baby and administer a feeding. The most obvious consideration is volume. While it might make sense to whip up bottles of formula on an as-needed basis for a singleton, this approach won't do with two hungry babies potentially headed toward meltdown. You need to be prepared.

## Making Enough Formula

Our approach was to make a huge batch of formula for the next day before going to bed at night. We lined up the bottles in the fridge in the same manner and location that we had lined up beers in our former life. We tried to have the number we anticipated using the next day ready, and depending on where we were in the nursing/comping/bottle-feeding continuum, the number of bottles could be anywhere from two to twenty. Though you'll get used to it shortly, the whole process is a pain in the butt. Baby formula clumps when it mixes, which is just so unfair. Even crueler, you can't use hot water to mix it. If you are worried about the purity of the water you are using and want to boil it first, you will need to boil it and then cool it to room temperature before you use it. We eventually had huge vats of bottled water sitting on the kitchen counter at room temperature, at the ready to mix with formula.

It is better to make lots of bottles of half servings than to throw out unfinished formula if a bottle goes unfinished. So measure the bottles on the short side and just pull out another one if one of your little snarfers does a particularly good job at a feeding. Bear in mind that formula has a very short refrigerator shelf life that varies from brand to brand but should be taken seriously. Normally, this window is between twenty-four to forty-eight hours, maximum. So the plan you were just hatching to buy a refrigerator for the basement and prepare 617 bottles every Sunday evening won't work. Newborns usually take about two to three ounces every two or three hours, so start by making two-ounce servings. Eventually, you will be making eight-ounce bottles, but not for many months.

The goals at any stage are never to have to make a baby wait long while you prepare a bottle and never to waste formula, because it's expensive. Don't let that expense tempt you to toss a half-used bottle back into the fridge, however, as bacteria grow quickly on and in them. Definitely not worth the risk. Once a baby's mouth touches a bottle, the formula either goes into the baby or down the drain. The bottom line on preparing bottles is that even if you don't have the energy or foresight to prepare every serving for the next day, you absolutely want to have enough ready to get you through the night and the morning's first feed. When a baby wakes up hungry, neither of you will enjoy the time it takes you to mix a bottle of formula.

## Bottle Warmers

I have already pooh-poohed bottle warmers on the belief that a pan of hot water is a great three-minute warmer-to-perfection of baby bottles. If you must have the warmer, go for it. Do not, however, be tempted to use the microwave to warm bottles. If the reports of leaching carcinogens from heated plastic aren't enough to scare you off, then the prospect of scalding your little darlings' palates ought to at least give you pause. Yes, the microwave oven is fast and convenient, but it heats inconsistently and it's just too hard to judge temperature safely by simply squirting your wrist. A pan of hot water worked well for grandma and still does today, but please, please don't pop the bottle into the pan and then put it on the stove. The pan method involves simply boiling water, pulling the pan from the stove, and *then* putting the bottle in the water for a few minutes. It only requires that you anticipate a feeding by more than a few minutes, which you will do readily within a week or two. For those that sneak up on you, even an upset baby can make it a few minutes to mealtime as you hold him and talk to him, reassuring him that it's coming.

## Reality Check

An enduring memory I have of the first year of my babies' lives is standing at the end of the day in front of a sink piled up with bottles, exhausted and drawing a deep breath in order to start preparations for the next day. At the beginning, we were determined to sterilize every bottle perfectly in a lobster pot of boiling water. Within a few weeks, we were popping them in the dishwasher. In order to have them ready for the before-bed preparation of the next day's bottles, this had to happen around dinnertime...either that, or we would have needed to purchase about thirty bottles so that we could use previously cleaned ones. It wouldn't be a bad idea, if you can resign yourself to the expense. There are so many different bottles on the market now, however, that it wouldn't make sense to buy dozens of any particular brand until your babies have tried a few different sorts. As the owners of two gassy little guys, we preferred the fancy Dr. Brown's that magically pushed the air to the back of the milk. They cost more per unit than our crystal wedding glasses and had about fifteen parts each that all needed to be cleaned. We didn't care, because the boys really seemed more comfortable after drinking from them than from others. With our non-gassy first child, the squat Avent bottles with the wide nipple base were great. More recently, some parents are going back to glass baby bottles, in order to allay their worries about the possible risk of leaching BPA (bisphenol A) in plastic bottles. In any case, try a few types out for each baby before buying fifty of anything.

### Other Considerations

Just as one does when breastfeeding, you'll want to be sure to run to the bathroom to pee before beginning to feed your babies. Pop the bottles in a pan of hot water, make your trip to the restroom (surely

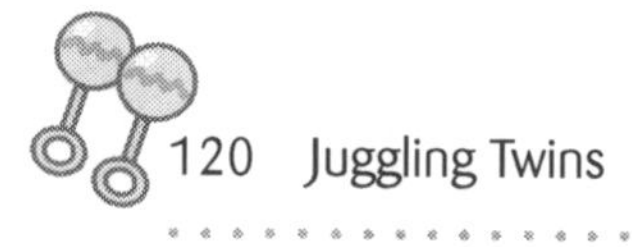


you know how to pee with a baby in your arms by now), and by the time you wash and return, the bottles will be nearly ready. If you intend to feed them together, you will need to learn some of the same juggling tricks nursing moms do and will perhaps want to invest in a double nursing pillow or two Boppy pillows. Feeding them at the same time will take some practice, and in particular, it will take time for you to learn the art of burping one while continuing to feed the other. Babies get justifiably enraged when they are suckling happily only to have the nipple ripped from their lips. Saying, "Just a minute, I have to burp your brother" likely won't do much to quell the screaming.

While you may feel confident handling the babies with one hand each, it's a trick that's not without its dangers. If you are certain you want to try, be sure to surround yourself with pillows and consider swaddling the babies tightly before the feeding so that you have more control over their necks and heads as you move them to your shoulder. It is possible to bottle feed both of them in your lap at once and it will become easier to do so as they get older.

Similarly to the breastfeeding scenario, however, it makes a lot of sense to feed each of them separately in the first weeks, so that you can observe and bond with each of them individually. A Boppy pillow next to you can help you keep one baby happy and safe from the danger of rolling away as she waits her turn to eat or relaxes after a bottle. Eventually, you will be able to feed them simultaneously, with each propped on a Boppy pillow on either side of you. Tandem feedings will soon be a snap, and you are only months away from propping the babies in bouncy seats, handing them their bottles, and watching in awe as they pop them in their own mouths happily.

# 13 On Schedule or On Demand?

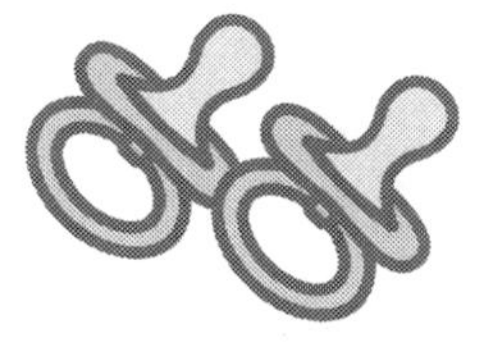

When my eldest was a newborn, her intermittent crying rattled me to the point that I sought the advice of a mother of four who lived across the street. "She's probably hungry," she said. "Just feed her more."

"No," I said. "That can't be it. It happens sometimes when she has eaten only two hours previously." The woman just stared at me, a bit dumbfounded. Then she laughed.

"Just feed her," she repeated, now smiling patiently.

I did. It worked. The poor kid was hungry. It turns out I had been a bit too literal in my interpretation of the baby how-to books when I had read that babies eat every three hours. It hadn't been three hours, so she couldn't be hungry, right? But mine seemed to want to eat all the time...at least that week. The next week, it changed. We tried at that point to listen to the baby more and not be too wedded to a plan. It began to seem that babies aren't terribly respectful of plans. At that point in my parenting, the idea of trying to get a newborn on a prefabricated eating schedule was looking both unrealistic and misguided. I decided babies should have the privilege, as we do, of eating when they are hungry, which can be anywhere from every thirty minutes to every three hours.

However, I can now tell you with some authority that with twins, practicing on-demand feeding will pretty much kill you. I don't mean a slow, painful death; it shouldn't take long at all, really. Here's the thing: *everything is different with twins!* By its nature, on-demand feeding is a system without a schedule, and it will be very difficult indeed to keep this ship afloat with no schedule whatsoever. Call me archaic if you need to; I can take it. But I have the support of every overnight twin nanny and multiples specialist I know to back me up here. Working at every stage to create a semblance of a schedule will create a more tranquil, predictable, manageable household for these babies, and the fact is that they will not starve. I promise. This is not a call to "stretch them" cruelly to the next feeding as they howl lamentably in hunger. The plan is simply to attempt to build three-hour cycles in the day: a blueprint with which one starts this project every morning, that states what to expect—or hope for, anyway—for its duration. Yes, there may be deviations, but the key is to start with a design for the day and to gently, steadily guide the babies towards compliance.

Structure is something all children absolutely crave. Structure and predictability give kids security. I believe this need for order starts young—very young—and never really goes away. If our need for order ever really went away, those giant chain stores that specialize in plastic boxes for us to put all our things in wouldn't be making bazillions of dollars a year selling us the false hope of an ordered life. You've already paid them for stackable boxes with sliding drawers for the babies' stuff, haven't you? Return the boxes and commit to a feeding schedule instead! Without a schedule, you will simply be a disordered person with a lot of plastic boxes in her house.

By the time our kids were three months old, we were following a very reliable schedule, and this was absolutely the key to our sanity. It allowed us to predict their needs in a manner that made our self-scheduling of coverage more manageable, and it contributed in incalculable ways to the general calm of the household. We warmed bottles five minutes before the babies knew they were hungry; we knew when they were likely to wake from naps, stage a meltdown, or need a walk; we could see the day in front of us every morning and pretty much know what it would demand of us. If these reasons

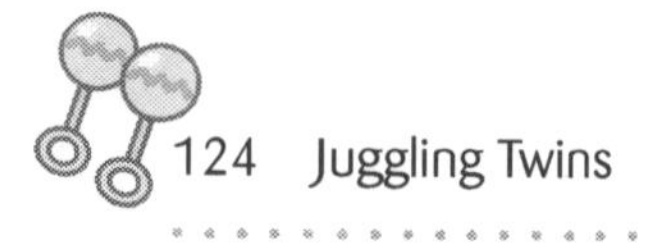


aren't compelling for you, try this one: *we got more sleep.* In fact, we eventually got plenty of it, all because of the work we put in on the front end to begin to establish a schedule that was in place when they were developmentally able to get through the night. And eventually, they did. And we slept.

## Establishing a Feeding Schedule

If your babies are at least five to six pounds, you can begin to create a daily feeding plan that will, by the time they are seven pounds, begin to resemble a schedule of sorts. At this stage, nighttime is still an on-demand free-for-all, so this proposal doesn't discuss feedings between 10 p.m. and 6 a.m. While you can (and should) organize the adults' nighttime responsibilities and shifts, you cannot hope to have the babies on an eating schedule per se during the night. The "schedule" begins in the morning, and the challenge is to keep it going as long as you can, with the goal of making it to a 10 p.m. feeding with everyone intact, including you.

Normally, babies cooperate with this strategy beautifully by waking fairly dependably around 6 a.m., regardless of the level of overnight hooliganism they have wrought upon the household. And guess what I'm suggesting you do if they don't wake up on their own then? Yep...just what you may have heard you never should do: wake them up. (Twins are different! You can let your *next* kid sleep 'til noon.) Yes, I realize that the concept of setting an alarm in order to get up and wake two sleeping babies sounds absolutely absurd. But keep your eyes on the prize! This is about long-term, truly meaningful, delayed gratification, which is to say that if you can get the family into this proposed rhythm, you're going to have a chance at full nights of sleep in three months. So fight your impulse to throw something—probably this book—at the alarm; get up and get them going with the first feeding. Sadly, if you are reading this while you are still pregnant, you don't yet realize that you'll probably be up already anyway. Even on their most active nights, babies don't *sleep in* the way you used to after an active night—they'll probably be awake anyway and your alarm clock probably won't get even remotely involved.

So the day begins with a 6 a.m. feeding, and from there the idea is to try to make it to 9 a.m., then noon, then 3 p.m., then 6 p.m., and then *not* 9 p.m. but instead to 10 p.m. Generally, the first three feedings will best follow your plan. If you are breastfeeding, you have the most milk to offer during this time frame, and the babies are more likely to feel "settled" afterwards, as they have had hours of dark, quiet time overnight to detox from all of yesterday's stimulation. But by 6 p.m., young babies in particular are overstimulated by all they have heard and seen that day and are usually threatening meltdown. Bear in mind that being alive is pretty stimulating to them at this point—it doesn't take a trip to an amusement park. *Everything* is new, and the collective newness is understandably overwhelming. Try to imagine how you would feel at the end of a long day on Venus. Cranky and tired, no? A nursing baby is also dealing with a diminishing return on nursing efforts, as your supply at this time of day is at its lowest point. You should be flexible, obviously.

The overarching goal, of course, is to keep everyone in one piece; maintaining a schedule is always secondary. Whatever shape the schedule retains after that 3 p.m. feeding, however, one habit that is truly worth establishing is a 10 p.m. feeding or, at minimum, a top-off (even if there has been a feeding within the previous hour). In an ideal world, you will never see this feeding—you will only hear about it, as you will be going to sleep shortly after the 6 p.m. feeding and will sleep until one of the babies awakens between 1 a.m. and 3 a.m. If you are breastfeeding and you are awake at this time, cluster feeding (nursing in short, repeated sessions) on demand from 6–10 p.m. is a good idea, and it won't preclude that 10 p.m. feeding, believe it or not.

## Reality Check

It was an overnight twin nanny who established this feeding schedule for us, and we complied readily once we saw its benefits. We were certainly rewarded for our efforts when the babies more or less started sleeping through at about twelve weeks. Generally, the 6 a.m. feeding felt to us like a "reboot"; it initiated the schedule for the day, and from there hell was free to loose itself upon us but generally didn't. The 10 p.m. feeding was less psychologically beneficial and more practical: "topping them off" at 10 p.m. was crucial in moving them toward sleeping through the night. Even at very early stages, it made their night sleeping more settled and assured. Again, even if they had eaten at 9 p.m., we topped them at 10 p.m. before heading to bed. In the early weeks, we considered making it from 10 p.m. until 1 a.m. to be a good stretch, and expected to be up again with them around 4 a.m.; by three months, though, they were making it through to 6 a.m. We credit the 10 p.m. top-off and three-hour rotations during the day with getting them there. And yes, for those middle-of-the night feedings when one woke to eat, we woke the other, too.

Waking the second baby to eat is yet another episode of truly having to fight one's instinct. You will *not* want to wake a slumbering child, and I certainly don't blame you. But it is much better to do two longish feeding sessions than four shorter ones, and a baby who has been awakened to eat is likely to return to a deep sleep relatively easily after being fed and changed.

Philosophically, it can be so tempting to choose a baby-driven, on-demand method of feeding that simply responds to an infant's needs. I assure you, I am generally a pro-baby sort of gal. In fact, not only do I like babies, but I also have a lot of respect for them. So I do get the whole concept of on-demand feeding. But hear me now, believe me later: coaxing your babies toward a schedule is not just to your advantage. They, too, will benefit from the ultimate nirvana the schedule seeks: full nights of sleep for everybody. And the host of additional benefits extends well beyond the obvious, as not only will they be happier kids once they nail down that skill, but they will also be in the possession of saner parents who can better cope with all the other challenges of nurturing two babies.

## Stay Flexible

No matter how thoughtful or deliberate your feeding decisions, you will need to be amenable to changing them utterly and quickly. Having that willingness to revisit a plan, break it down, and start again instantly has carried over to every best-laid plan we've hatched since. Determined to nurse both of our boys exclusively for a full year, I was at first sluggish to admit that it wasn't going well and that they needed complementary bottles. When I couldn't express enough milk for comps, we had to introduce some formula. When one of them subsequently struggled with the formula, we had to experiment with soy formulas. We combined breastfeeding and bottle with each, then tried breast with one, bottle with the other. I pumped, then I didn't. I obsessed. I organized and reorganized our plan for *who* would be eating *what*. And finally, we realized that no one strategy was going to see us through in a regular fashion, day in, day out.

The twins were constantly evolving, my supply was in flux, their needs were changing, and their capabilities were growing and emerging. What didn't work one week did the next, and vice versa. I had to learn to be less controlling and more responsive to their actual needs, both those demonstrated and those requiring some interpretation. As with every aspect of having two, we had to learn to be ready for anything. It was a good lesson to learn before they became toddlers, so that today, when I hear a harmonized "Uh oh!" from the other room, I can still tap into that sense of being prepared for anything and, when I walk in the room to find a gallon of olive oil pouring onto the rug—*glug, glug, glug*—I can quickly see that the scheduled playdate that morning might need to be postponed.

Here's an example of how not to get locked into a plan that might need tinkering: the hospital sends us all home with a few cans of formula (more if we think to sweet-talk the nurse). Without even giving it a conscious thought, we begin to view that brand of formula as carrying the blessing of neonatal experts. But the truth is that you may simply be given the brand made by the pharmaceutical company with the most money—the one best positioned to forge a deal with the hospital. Their gift to you does not mean this is the best formula for your babies; it may only mean that they did some promising research on Ebola in 2002 that sent their stock price soaring, giving them enough cash reserves to launch a plan to get their baby formula into the nurseries of urban hospitals in your area. So when the pediatrician suggests that your baby's potential reflux might be quelled by switching brands, you need to be flexible enough to give it a try. Certainly whatever work you do to increase your adaptability will help you not only this month but in the next hundred or so, because *everything's different with twins.*

# 14

# Coping with the Nights (To Sleep, Perchance to Scream...)

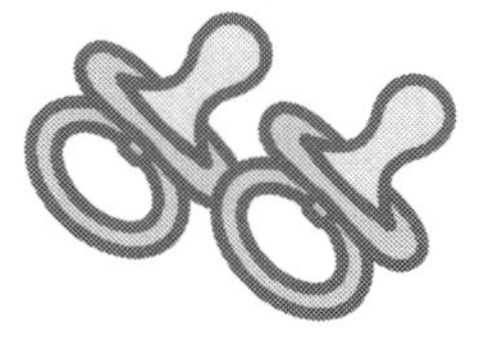

This is what they are talking about when you are pregnant. Your mother and sister, as they secretly talk about you over the phone. Your colleagues, as they watch you waddle to the restroom yet again. Your neighbors, peeking from behind their living room curtains as you rock yourself out of your car. "She has no idea," they murmur to each other, shaking their heads. It's not the feeding of, the paying for, the fights between, the teenage angst of, or the college tuition for your twins that's fretting them. It's your sleep. All of them remember vividly those nights when they haunted their own homes, specterlike, in the wee hours. Then they calculate the *doubled* lost sleep, and suddenly their knees get shaky at the thought, and they have a sudden urge to lie down on the floor in your honor. "Poor thing," they cluck. "She has absolutely no idea."

But you *do* have some idea, don't you? It actually *has* occurred to you, while you're lying awake in the middle of the night, your belly now the vast gymnasium in which your babies are conducting an impromptu floor exercise competition, that these kids are just as likely to be awake during the night once they are *outside* you as they are now, inside you. Of *course* you have an idea, if for no reason other than that you are not an utter idiot, and only an utter idiot would fail to see that, yes, taking care of two infants could in fact prove to be a challenge in any *number* of ways that would seem to include some sleep-scarcity issues.

Let's put this doomy-gloomy sleep deprivation talk into some context, shall we? Most people—grown-up people, anyway—are totally wacko about their sleep and hoard and guard it as a kid with ten siblings does her Halloween candy. Parents think back on their lost sleep with a sense of nostalgic heroism (their own) for their having done for a few months what firefighters, convenience store clerks, and nurses have been doing routinely forever—simply remaining awake while others in their age group are sleeping. Now, in the spirit of full disclosure, I confess that, when asked what I want for Christmas, I will reliably say "more shut-eye" every year. I do understand the impulse to protect one's precious sleep time with a certain ferociousness. And it is true, for several reasons, that you will at times be getting less sleep than anyone who is not a vampire would find feasible. The problem is really a logistical one. First, let's take a look at the facts.

## How Newborns Sleep. And Don't.

In spite of their appalling reputation and contrary to the incessant warnings you may get from friends who are parents—or in spite of what you remember, if this isn't your first round—babies actually sleep a lot. I mean *a lot* a lot. As in, they sleep more hours per day than you did when you were in college, even including the week during sophomore year when you got dumped and your roommates nursed you back to emotional stability by bringing you thirty-ounce wine coolers with a large straw every couple of hours for five days. More sleep than that.

Though every infant is of course different, the vast majority of them will actually sleep more than sixteen hours a day. So that's not the problem. The problem is the manner in which they get these sixteen hours. Newborns tend to bundle their sleep into inopportune little two-to-three hour *siestas* that typically happen more reliably during the day than at night. Initially, they are not able to string together more than a few hours in one stretch, and when they eventually do, they tend at first to do it not at night, like a reasonable person, but during the middle of the day. Yes, this is a totally unacceptable approach that may jeopardize your nearly lifelong habit of sleeping at night. I understand this. Perhaps, however, it will help you be open-minded to newborns' chosen method of sleeping if you bear in mind two factors that make it impossible for them to see things your way at this early point in your relationship: their brains and their stomachs.

## It's Biological

Young babies' brains don't really perceive the difference between night and day as sharply as ours do, leading to the common assessment that babies "have their days and nights confused." A more precise explanation is that their pituitary glands don't yet release sufficient melatonin to regulate their circadian rhythms. As a result, their sleep is still "disorganized" at this early stage in the sense that the brain isn't yet effective at sending the body signals to sleep in regular patterns of extended, consolidated hours. I don't know about you, but this excuse gets a lot of mileage with me. In light of my own occasional managerial mishaps, I can't help but have a bit more empathy when the problem is described in terms of their less-than-perfect organizational skills. I get that.

The second biological challenge that leads to infant wakefulness is the size of their stomachs. Newly born babies need to eat at least every three hours. In this respect, it is actually not a good idea to let a baby sleep more than a few hours at a time in the early weeks, as that pretty much means he or she has skipped a meal. Until a baby weighs seven pounds, she should be fed closer to every two hours; at seven pounds, she may make it to three. If you are breastfeeding, your babies will digest your milk more quickly than they would formula, so your babies are likely to be on the short end of the predicted range of sleep periods. Furthermore, if your babies were preemies, it's possible that your pediatrician wants them fed at much shorter intervals. In this context, you may be able to forgive your twins for sleeping in less-than-ideal lumps of time. It's not just that they're not ready to do so; it wouldn't even be healthy for them to do so just yet. They need to eat.

## Reality Check

Be forewarned that there is always one mother at the playground who will smile placidly at the baby in her stroller while announcing that "he's really an easy baby...he's already sleeping though the night," when you know for a fact that the child is so young that the woman is still wearing pants that have an elastic panel at the front. Don't be alarmed. First of all, she's probably lying. If not, then what she really means by "through the night" is that they slept through his crying the other night and eventually the baby fell back asleep without eating. Bear in mind that she is also the mother who will later be telling you that her kid is doing phonics when yours is out-of-her-head proud when she stacks three blocks into a tower. If it helps, you can feel very confident that she paid big, this braggart, because the hour after that "through the night" stretch was likely a nightmare of famished, manic meltdown from which it was difficult for her baby to return.

At this age, babies need to wake up to eat every three hours, maximum, and it should console you to know that waking and feeding a newborn who sleeps more than three hours, painful as it is to you, is the beginning of establishing the schedule that will lead you back to sanity.

As suggested in the previous chapter, your "schedule" will operate in two-to-three hour cycles that will normally have your babies waking twice to eat during the night. Yes, twice *each*. And again, the idea is that when one baby wakes to eat, she is changed, fed, burped, and returned to bed, and if this process has not awakened her twin, then *you* will, in order to keep them on parallel programs. Thus, the nightly sleep that you have come to expect will be twice interrupted by two rather involved feeding sessions of more than an hour. On a good night.

An ugly picture, indeed, but let's keep our heads, shall we?

### The Good News

1. As it turns out, a night of lost or scattered sleep will not kill you. If it did, the bodies of medical residents and 7-Eleven managers would be strewn all over the streets of our cities at every sunrise.
2. The cumulative effect of too little sleep won't kill you, either. Even parents of higher-order multiples—triplets and more—don't die of exhaustion. Not right away, anyway.
3. This is a truly temporary situation, to be endured for a matter of weeks. Okay...quite a few weeks. But weeks, not years. This is not forever. You can do anything for a while, as long as you have an end in sight, right? The problem is that because you don't know when it will end, it doesn't quite feel temporary. It is. I promise.
4. Unlike other exhausted people, you will be allowed and even encouraged to take naps. Most Americans now consider napping an absurd indulgence. This is because we can't multitask while napping, other than to have sex while asleep...which actually happens to be another skill you will be perfecting soon. In any case, you, unlike most of us, will be instantly forgiven when you take a little break from dinner to lay your heavy head down gently on the cozy, warm slice of meat loaf on your plate to doze off for a spell. "She had no idea," they will coo, as they tenderly wipe gravy from your ear whorls. "She should really get some sleep."
5. Say! Did we mention that this doesn't last forever?

## The Not-So-Secret Weapons

In spite of these consolations, getting yourself and your partner through the first weeks and months of caring for newborns poses true challenges, many of them related to your own mounting fatigue. Even in the best-case scenario—when you have a plan, *and* the adults in the house are all on board, *and* the babies in the house are only melting down in the expected ways, rather than in constant, inconsolable, or arbitrary ways—*even then,* you are going to feel simply wrecked much of the time. If you insist on pursuing the worst-case scenario—muddling through with a schedule-less, triage-based strategy of "we'll just see what happens"—your exhaustion will be monstrous; your ability to cope, negligible. While working toward a schedule is the obvious, overarching goal for avoiding constant household uproar and distress, having some simple, trusty tools and techniques for settling babies will provide the moment-to-moment relief essential for everybody's sanity. Some of the best ideas for helping upset babies back to a state of calm are not new at all. In fact, they're ancient.

## Swaddling

Full-length books have been written with the sole purpose of advocating the practice of swaddling babies. Let me save you some time here. They are absolutely right, but you needn't read an entire history of the practice of baby-wrapping among primeval peoples to be convinced of this, fascinating as it is. Here's the basic premise, as I understand it: as we ever so gradually evolved from furry knuckle-scrapers into a people who could simultaneously drive and manipulate the toggle wheel on an iPod, our skulls grew bigger in order to encase our swelling cerebella and cerebra, which have needed more and more room to hold the names of all our favorite playlists.

So while the evolving human body has stayed on the small, apish side, the head slowly did a Charlie Brown sort of thing, getting increasingly large relative to the body underneath it. This meant that the ratio of a fetus's head size to its mom's pelvis was becoming less and less favorable to the mom. At this point, the evolutionary process had a decision to make: either rip women to shreds and perhaps make both them and their fledgling offspring extinct in the collective process of getting all those Charlie Browns out, or get Charlie Brown out sooner, when his head isn't quite so large. Though mothers in labor might swear in the moment that evolution chose the former, it actually seems to have chosen the latter, and purportedly began releasing babies from their gestation earlier—eventually, about three months earlier—than the year it ought to take them to develop, all in order to fit that big head through the birth canal.

Those who espouse this theory suggest as evidence our utter incompetence as infants, compared to other species. They note that when other animals are born, they unceremoniously get up, trot around the barnyard, and say "Howdy do" to their new neighbors, whereas we mostly squawk and blink, alarmed at our sudden *ex utero* situation. It's not just that we fail to lick ourselves off and get up to go for a stroll. We're entirely dependent on our parents for *everything*. In fact, we're so thoroughly inept, having been pushed from our fetal status before being fully cooked, that we hardly even know how to go to sleep without some help. So says this theory, and I must say that spending some time with newborns does lend anecdotal support to the notion that these little guys would be much happier back where they were. Just about everything appears to overwhelm, threaten, and exhaust them, unlike their equine counterparts, who are signed up for galloping lessons on day two.

Basically, for the first three months of their lives, babies are longing only to be back in the womb. Doesn't that just make sense? Doesn't their every fuss, squall, and squirm seem to be saying, "Where did that womb go?" If my scientific hypothesizing hasn't yet convinced you, then the reaction that you get when you first properly swaddle a baby will.

Swaddling is essentially the practice of recreating with a blanket or wrap the same secure immobility that the baby was accustomed to in the womb. By virtually binding them in a fixed position, you are returning them to a state of familiar refuge, where their limbs can't flail beyond their control and they are encased cocoonlike in a protective wrap. Baby twins seem even more responsive to the comfort of swaddling and maybe, just maybe, this is because they are that much more smooshed than the average singleton *in utero*. All I know is what I've seen, and I have seen swaddling work some bona fide miracles on screaming twins.

Proper technique in swaddling requires faith. In order to achieve the desired effect, one must believe, for example, in the basic impossibility of squeezing a child to death with a square patch of cotton. The first time I swaddled one of my crying babies, I wrapped him the same way I did my dolls when I was seven years old: I placed him down on a blanket, flipped the ends over each other loosely, and then scooped the whole bundle up like a small load of delicate washables. "No, no, no, no," said the twin nanny, shoving me aside with a hip-check and grabbing the bundle to show me how it should be done. In four seconds flat, she expertly arranged the blanket with geometric precision, placed him in it just so, and then performed what appeared to be an elaborate origami trick, culminating in her *cinching* my precious child so tightly that I fully expected to see his esophagus squirt out of his mouth. I stood with my hands over my mouth and my eyebrows raised to my hairline, unable to speak my horror. But at the same instant, he hushed and his eyes seemed to glaze over in a state of detached bliss. I was traumatized, but he was perfectly placated.

## Reality Check

It took me days to be able to create the cinching effect our nanny had, but I did finally get it, and the comfort that tightness engendered once I got it taut enough built my confidence that this was a practice

*continued…*

the babies would benefit from rather than something that would get them placed quickly into suitable foster homes. It became clear that they were helped by it when they were repeatedly quieted by the procedure, often falling asleep shortly after being wrapped. On the blessed nights that we had overnight help, we would get up in the morning to find the babies side by side in bouncy seats at a 45 degree incline, each wrapped liked an impervious burrito, so stiff that we could have picked them up and carried them at our sides like schoolbooks without disturbing them...and both of them sleeping blissfully. We wanted to salute them, their rigid little bearings were so taut. (Instead, we saluted the nanny—*O Captain! My captain!*)

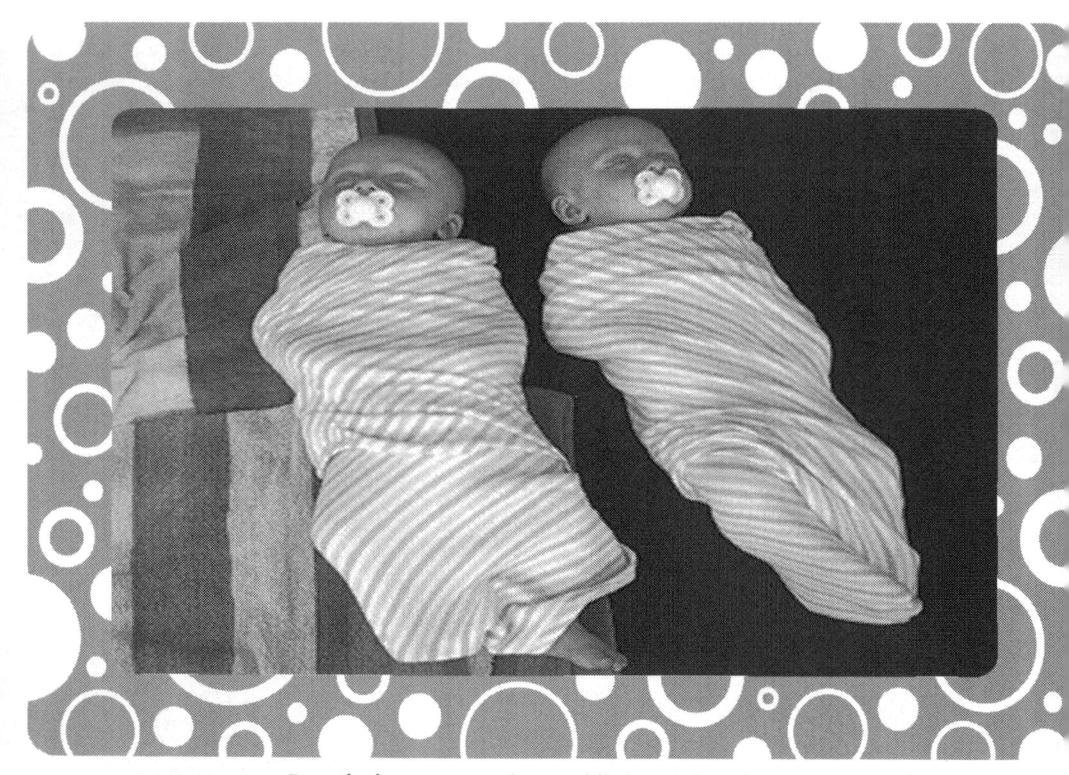

Even if a foot escapes, the swaddle keeps them happy.

Photo courtesy of the Regan-Loomls family

Good, effective swaddling demands the perfect blanket. Clever marketers now sell baby wraps of various materials for just this purpose, with an assortment of binding methods. Word on Twin Street is that these are worthwhile for some kids, but they aren't cheap, and you'll certainly need more than one for each baby. We had ten cotton blankets and still found ourselves hunting for clean ones now and then, as we happened to be experiencing a bit of a production slow-down in our laundry room at this point. You will likely get a few receiving blankets as gifts, but not all of these will necessarily be useful as swaddling blankets. In the first place, a swaddling blanket must be made of breathable cotton. Do not use fleece or flannel for swaddling babies. As if suffocation and overheating aren't threat enough, flannel and fleece don't stretch, so there's no way to achieve the perfect cinch with them. Don't even use these blankets *around* young babies. They are not as breathable as knit cotton and so pose safety issues if a baby's face is ever covered or, more likely, if the baby becomes overheated. Find blankets with that thin, stretchy waffle-weave cotton that your long underwear was made of when you were a kid. We were able, with light knit cotton blankets, to swaddle our babies right through the summer without once overheating them. The right cotton blanket will stretch as you pull it and should not be much bigger than three feet across.

To create the perfect swaddle, lay a square blanket down with one corner at the top (so that the blanket looks like a diamond). Fold the top corner down to about the middle of the square; don't bring it all the way to the opposite corner, however. Place the baby on it so that her shoulders are level with the fold you have just made. Pull the left corner over her body, and use the side of your hand to hold it in place against her left side as you pull the remaining material out from under her to the right, stretching it until it's taut. Only after it is tight should you bring the right corner across the top. The bottom bits can either flap loosely or get tucked up before that final fold of

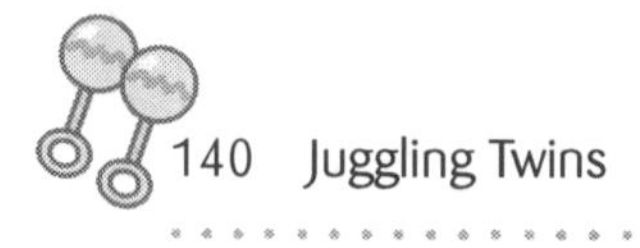


the right corner happens. It's that pulling on the right corner while your hand holds the blanket in place against the baby that creates the desired effect, so that's the most important step to get right. As you practice, note that pulling tightly does not hurt the child and may in fact be the exact moment she calms down.

## A Womb with a View: Other Methods to Encourage Sleep

Whether or not we are aware of the fact, our instinctual methods of helping a baby sleep are all rough approximations of life in the womb. Rocking a baby simulates the sway of a mother's walk while pregnant, for example, and *shush*ing recreates the sounds of the womb. These techniques are so well established in our DNA that when a baby cries as her mother waits in line at the grocery store, all the women around them sway together like a field of tall grass in the wind. When your baby is disconcerted, the more you can do to convince him that this is all a bad dream and he is actually still in the womb, the better your chances of calming him. In the middle of the night, with a baby who has been fed, changed, and swaddled but is still not happy, sometimes the best approach is to sit in a completely dark room and just hold him closely, on his side. Sometimes even rocking or walking are more stimulation than he needs, and simply lying in your arms will quiet him in ways that one couldn't have imagined when he was unraveling.

Less instinctual but more addictive is the use of pacifiers. Our über-parenting of child number one (no pacifiers!) was turned on its head for numbers two and three when the hospital staff popped giant pacifiers in their mouths and seemed to imply that we were cruel if we intended to remove them before their seventh birthday. The calming effect was clear enough, and we relented before we even got them home, because we knew we wouldn't always be able to offer each of them the quieting techniques we had offered their older sister—at least not in a timely fashion. The pacifiers became our good friends during the first three months, not just at night but also when a baby was waiting his turn to be fed.

Some parents swear by white-noise machines that recreate the roar of the womb and block out the neighbors' arguments. You can spend a pile of cash on elaborate ones from gadget stores at the mall, or you can use the kind we did: a household fan. If that's not enough noise, put a radio in the room with the dial between stations; the static works well for some babies.

## Co-Sleeping

The practice of co-sleeping—that is, the family bed scenario in which the whole gang sleeps like a heap of contented puppies and the parents never have sex until the kids are eleven and have finally been convinced to get their own dang beds—is in my opinion a laughable proposition for families with twin babies. But then, I'm prone to inappropriate laughter, so please take no offense if you insist on trying to put both babies between you every night. The tender scenes described in the books that tell us how to sleep with children in our beds (leading one to wonder just how complicated it can be) are, like everything else, different with twins. In the first place, you had better have at least a queen-sized bed; full Parliament is preferable.

Secondly, wave goodbye to that spouse on the other side of the bed. You just gave up the only five minutes of daily intimacy you have been allotted. Admittedly, there are compelling reasons for this practice, all of them very appealing to my sense that babies deserve as much comfort as we can provide them. But logistics interfere once more. There are simply a lot of you now, and you're going to be interrupting each other's sleep in ways that you won't be if everyone has his or her own sleeping arrangements.

For example: babies sleep like pigs. I don't mean that they always lie snuggled side by side and appear to be smiling. I mean they snort like pigs. Sleeping babies make loud, wheezy, raspy barnyard noises that aren't exactly snoring but function just like snoring in that they keep others awake. It's hard enough to relax while listening to this on a monitor; having two of them snarfling in person all night right next to you will be downright alarming. Whenever we co-slept with our oldest, the quality of my sleep was always *off,* as there was a constant hum in my head—a sort of unconscious little tune that went "don't-smoosh-baby, don't-smoosh-baby, don't-smoosh-baby."[1] And to this day, when our kids scamper to our bed seeking refuge from the ghoulish nightmares nipping at their heels, I awake the next morning stiff and cranky, having slept in a physics-defying perch from which half my back side has been draped off the bed. But perhaps you're a better sleeper or a better person than I and will seize the co-sleeping opportunity as a time for precious bonding. Let me know how that goes.

## Cribs

If you decide to sleep your kids in cribs, you will only need one for the two of them at any given moment for a number of months. Our babies never woke each other with crying at this age—they always slept through it in that astonishing way newborn babies have of sleeping through everything short of sonic booms. Because they were swaddled, they couldn't kick each other awake, either. Ours shared a crib until they were four months old.

---

1. Co-sleeping is variously cited as potentially causing SIDS and as potentially reducing its incidence. Be sure to research this controversial question to your satisfaction before making any decisions about co-sleeping.

Most often, you will be putting babies down shortly after they have eaten, which makes it essential that you not put them down flat if they are to sleep well. Because the muscle at the base of the esophagus is still developing, babies need to be put down at an incline in order to digest their food comfortably. Not surprisingly, they will sleep better this way, which is why so many babies end up doing a lot of their sleeping in car seats on the living room floor or in bouncy seats or swings. They fall asleep well in those spots in part because their digestion is aided by gravity, which helps keep the food where it belongs. You can create the same effect with cribs by putting the babies down across the mattress horizontally—that is, perpendicular to the way we normally sleep in beds—after stacking a few piles of magazines between the mattress and the crib bottom, under the side their heads occupy.[2]

This practice might eliminate the need for you to do what my cousin and his wife did with their twins, which was to get them to sleep in their car seats (you got it...by driving them around the block forty times) and then *put the car seats in the crib* in order to convince the babies, and perhaps themselves, that they were sleeping in a crib. We were somewhat quicker to admit that ours weren't quite in cribs yet when we unapologetically put them to sleep in bouncy seats for the entire first month. Though the seats are designed for older babies, we swaddled the babies and then strapped them in tightly with the bottom of the swaddle resting within the straps (no feet going through), and they slept beautifully.

By one month, however, they were sleeping in a crib with the mattress raised at about a ten or twenty degree angle. We used "wedges" to keep them positioned on their backs, but these may have been unnecessary, as the babies weren't going anywhere, mummified

2. Putting magazines under the mattress is safer than placing something under the crib legs, particularly if there are pets or other children in the home.

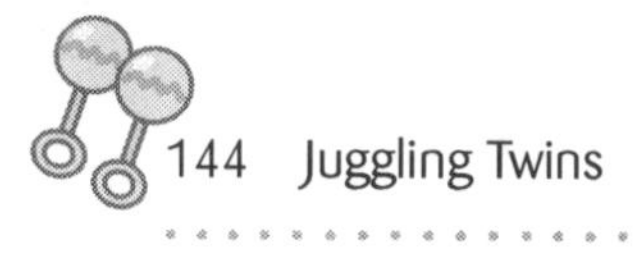


as they were in their swaddling blankets.[3] We sometimes snuggled them close to each other in a "spoon," but this never worked out quite as tenderly as our dreamy vision of this cozy scene promised. Though they surely were aware of each other at some subconscious level, they never appeared to acknowledge each other in the least for months.

## Getting Them Down

Newborn babies haven't yet developed that essential childhood skill of fighting sleep. In a matter of months, they will have it perfected and will begin employing it in earnest, stopping only after they complete graduate school. But at the moment, they are nearly helpless in the face of their own fatigue. Getting them to sleep is pretty much a matter of putting them down when they drift off. They probably won't protest if you put them in a crib after they have drifted off in your arms. This will not be the case a few months down the line, so if you're thinking that you just want to hold them as they sleep because they're so precious, bear in mind that there will be plenty of opportunities to do so in four months, and now might be a good time to do the laundry instead.

Establishing a routine before sleep is a good idea no matter how much of the concept they are absorbing in any obvious way. They will soon enough, and the routine will become like a narcotic if you are consistent with it. Ours was simple: change, swaddle, sway, sing, and down. The "sway" for us was what our friend Kathy calls the "chicken dance," wherein a parent, holding a swaddled baby, points both feet outward and bounces in an alternating fashion on each bent leg, two bounces per leg, for an effect not unlike an uncomfortable seventh-grade boy at his first dance. Doing this while singing would

---

3. The American Academy of Pediatrics strongly recommends that parents sleep their babies on their backs in order to help prevent SIDS.

be a real feat, so we generally separated the tasks. But each was very important to the process.

Years later, while we have dropped the chicken dance, we still sing the same lullaby before bed. We did make the mistake—okay, I made the mistake, fancying myself a latter-day Mary Poppins—to choose as our standard tune the "Stay Awake" lullaby that Mary sings to Jane and Michael Banks; suffice it to say you should not pick a song that only Julie Andrews can manage, with sudden minors or a C major that will hurt you and distress your audience. Regardless of the quality of our warbling, by the time the babies were six months old, we only needed to get to the third note before they became hypnotized and glazed over...though in retrospect I can see that they may have been faking in order to get us to stop singing.

## Break It into Shifts

Having methods for getting them to sleep is great, but it assumes that you only have one baby in your arms. So how does this work with two babies? Well, if you are following the previously outlined feeding schedule, you will be getting one down at a time. Their feedings will be slightly staggered, and thus the start of their sleep periods will be slightly staggered. That will help. But at this point, during this first month, the real answer is that you shouldn't be doing this alone. For the first month, your dream team should be operating in shifts at night, even if it hasn't established a shift formation during the day. If you have a third set of hands, as in your mother or mother-in-law or sister, you may possibly have three laborers to get you through the night, assuming your help is willing to do so. This is truly not a given, and you may feel that it is unfair to ask someone who is visiting in order to "help out" to start pulling all-nighters on your behalf. But hey...no harm in asking! I have permanently etched in my head the vision—and really, what a vision it was—of my dear sister stumbling down our hall in her fuzzy robe at 3 a.m. to report for duty, fumbling with her glasses and looking like she had just

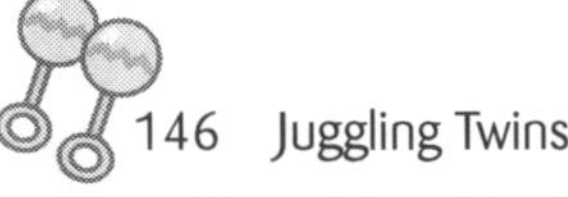


had her hair slammed in the car door. I adored her long before that night, but that moment sealed my devotion for eternity.

If your babies take bottles, either because they are fully formula-fed or because you are supplementing with formula, then it is crucial to break up the night into shifts. The first shift starts at 6:30 p.m. This is not your shift; in fact, you are required to go to bed now. This is because you are the only adult in the house—or on the block, for that matter—for whom sleeping at 6:30 p.m. is a totally plausible concept. The very latest you should be asleep in bed this month is 8 p.m. Seriously. The sleep that you get from 8 p.m. until the first wake-up call, around 2 a.m., is the only guaranteed sleep you get, so you must take it. Any sleep that happens after that is gravy. While you are asleep, someone else, preferably your partner, must handle the babies through the evening, including getting them their 10 p.m. bottles and popping them off to bed shortly thereafter. This means that you have to give up control of the ship so utterly that you are able to sleep with someone else at the helm. Go to bed, Ahab. They'll all be fine.

After the 10 p.m. feeding, everyone in the house should be asleep, until the first baby wakes up and you are on duty. If you happen to have an insomniac saint of a mother who is willing to take that second shift, *let her*. This is no time for manners. If you happen to have a trust fund, you will be spending most of it on an overnight baby nanny to handle this part of the fun. But if you're like most of us, it will be you who is getting up and playing ringleader to the circus that is in town from 2–6 a.m., grabbing sleep here and there between the wild animal acts. While you may need to wake up some adult reinforcements if both of the babies are coming unglued and you fear that you may be following them shortly, in general the idea is that one caretaker is on duty and one is sleeping. The coverage of the first morning shift, starting at 6 a.m., is negotiable. If you do have your mom or your sister in town, this is a reasonable shift for her to handle.

If not, it is fair to expect your partner to take this shift, also, while you grab another hour or two of rest. This may be an easier case to make if you point to the evidence that this is when the babies are on their best behavior and thus at the peak of their adorableness.

If you are nursing exclusively, it is unlikely in this first month that you have stockpiled enough expressed breast milk so that someone else can feed the babies while you sleep. You are probably in it for every feeding. The best way to get through the night in that situation is to approach every awakening as a team. That is, your helpers are responsible for going to the babies, changing them, bringing them to you, and then getting them back down once you have fed them. Your only job is to feed them. If you are able to nurse in bed, great, but if not, you should be in a darkened, comfy spot, where your singular responsibility is to nurse. Even in the absence of a schedule of shifts, you should try to go to bed at sunset. You will be grabbing sleep in small, unsatisfying chunks all night, and it takes a lot of them to resemble anything close to a passable night of rest. Eventually, even if you continue to nurse exclusively, you will have pumped enough breast milk that you will be able to sleep through the 10 p.m. feeding, which will afford you a solid stretch of sleep before the first wake-up call. Regardless of the elaborateness of the overnight help you have enlisted, you will not be able to sleep for a full eight hours even at that point, as your breasts would become engorged.

Given this picture, one can see why it is so helpful to have a third person involved during the first weeks, when the babies are still waking every few hours. Even if your partner is taking weeks off to help out, it makes a whole lot of sense to have a third set of hands until the babies are about eleven pounds. At that point, they will be capable of starting to stretch out their sleep to a much saner five hours, and that could—*could*—mean more sleep for everyone. That stage comes with its own sleep challenges, so help then will be a beautiful thing as well, but at the beginning, it is critical.

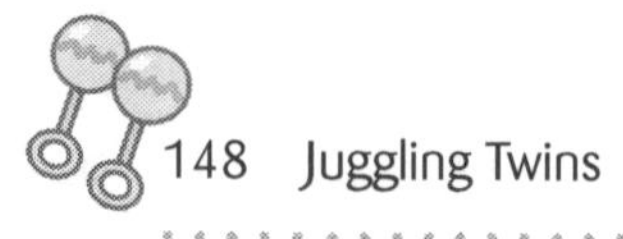



## You Are Not a Gullible Dolt

Remember: your babies cannot manipulate you. Even in their worst moments, all appearances to the contrary, they are not carrying out a systematic plot to exploit your goodwill. If a baby is awake and screaming, she means it. She is not arbitrarily testing the parameters of your patience or deviously keeping count of how many times you are willing to come to her. Bear in mind that one of the many things we tend to like about babies is that, the Doctrine of Original Sin notwithstanding, babies are purely innocent and therefore incapable of deception, cunning, or unsavory criminal activity. As complex as it can be to read them, babies themselves are not yet terribly complex, at least in terms of their needs. They need food, sleep, shelter, and comfort. If they cry, it is likely a lack of one of those things that is upsetting them. Hours of crying *may* stem from the discomfort of reflux, a stray pajama thread wound around her toe, or another "comfort" issue that is not entirely straightforward. But crying can never be interpreted as an attitude problem or a stubborn unwillingness to get along with one's new family.

You can be sure that, unlike adolescents or the peri-menopausal, babies cry for *reasons,* and the reasons can with some practice be ascertained. Even if you can't find a specific cause, most of their meltdowns can be attributed to being momentarily underfed or overwhelmed, and your first line of defense is always to address those issues calmly and methodically. Babies under three months are not cognitively ready to learn bad habits, so never hesitate to pick up a crying newborn because you fear spoiling him. You cannot. The purity of your relationship at this point is absolute: the babies have needs, and you can answer them. What could be simpler or more satisfying? Yes, yes, I know. Some sleep.

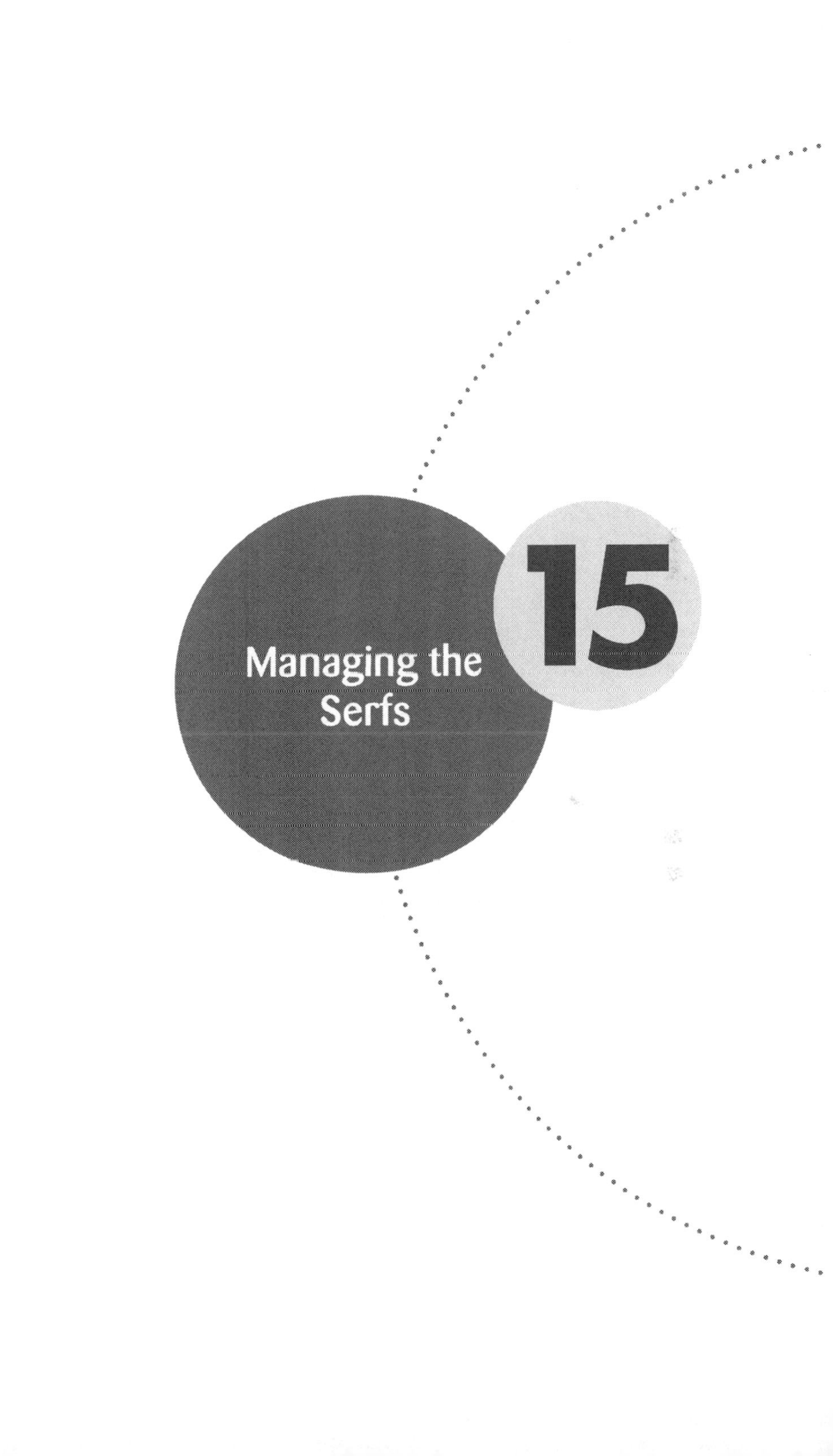

# 15 Managing the Serfs

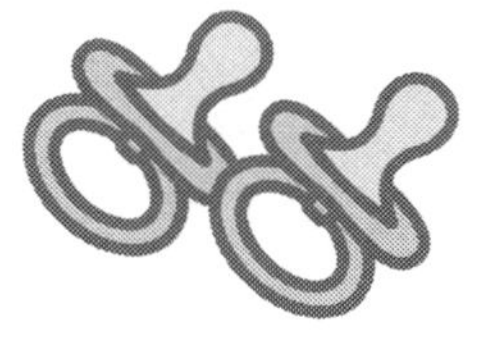

Anyone planning to come to see you and the babies in the first month should be warned that you now deem all visitors fair game for slave labor. More civilly, I suppose, a basic guideline for any guests in your home during the first month of your babies' lives is that they must provide more labor than their visit creates for the household. In truth, you ought to discourage visitations during the first month altogether in the hope that your babies can build up a little more immunity to their fellow humans' various bacteria and viruses before they are assaulted with them. But that's a bit unrealistic, probably, so this handy policy is the next best thing: you may come and gawk, but it will cost you.

The basic rate of entry to your home is a prepared meal that can be frozen; that should buy visitors about a twenty-minute stay. If they are not bringing a meal, then call before their visit to issue them a list of groceries that can be picked up on their way. Anyone arriving without food—a meal or a bagful—should absolutely be handed an assignment at the door. The most obvious tasks are folding a basket of clothes, taking an older sibling outside for some fresh air, watching the sleeping babies while you shower, walking the dog, watering the plants, or doing some dishes. These are not strenuous and can be accomplished in ten minutes or so; they should be doled out to people that you wouldn't mind seeing again. Save all suggestions about emptying diaper receptacles and scouring bathroom floors for those you'd be okay with not seeing again for a long while. If your guests need coffee, that's fine. They can make it and serve you some, too. And maybe throw a sandwich together for you while they're at it.

So how do you transition from being a courteous person with passable social skills to someone who nonchalantly hands her visitors a bucket and toilet brush as they enter her foyer? It's easier than you think! It turns out that this is just the first illustration of your seamless transformation from unassuming citizen to tribal chief. Duty-divvying is good training as you begin to take up your new position in your household as major domo, Mother Superior, clerk of the works...in short, as Queen of the Universe or at Least Your Corner of It. Look at me. I used to be a reasonably humble person, prone to apologizing before presuming to provide advice even to friends...and here I am ordering you around for hundreds of pages without a blush or even a clue as to who you are.

## Reality Check

Our babies were a couple of months old the first time my dear spouse gingerly suggested that I was getting a little bossy. My pithy response was something along the lines of, "Well, *duh.*" I always try to have clever responses like that one at the ready. This one was meant to synthesize the notions that (1) "I'm the Decider," as another alleged world leader has said. (2) Mama Bears *do* get bossy. Sorry. (3) No, actually I'm not. Sorry, that is. (4) Every team needs a captain and I voted for me; you missed the nomination process because it was held while you were at work. Which is where you are when I am *taking care of these babies all day!* (5) I have been hormonally rigged to rule this roost. It is really not so much a matter of choice as it is a glandular inevitability that neither of us is equipped to fight. (6) Give all of this some thought as you take the trash out, will you?

Again, there remains a good chance that you're a nicer person than I and that you will struggle in ways that I have not with the idea of marching well-meaning people—including the one you married—around at your bidding. In that case, you need to remember that most friends really do want to help, but need to be told how they can be most useful, and that most are especially happy to do so in ways that are not taxing or time consuming, as they assume they are still getting the same amount of credit they would have had they scrubbed your shower grout.

## How to Ask for Help

If you still have trouble asking for help directly, you can try one of several alternate passive-aggressive approaches:

- Sheepishly apologize for your pathetic neediness while handing over a list of chores. This approach acknowledges the abnormality of the request but preys upon their pity and results in their honoring it anyway.
- Find a deputy—a pushy friend who is in charge of doling out helpful tasks on your behalf, as if it were her idea. Everyone has at least one bossy-cow friend who would relish this role.
- Explain that your doctor has insisted that you need the help of friends. It's actually a medical necessity.
- Beg. Well up, choke up, butter up, break down. Whatever it takes.

By the third trimester of your pregnancy, you should already have lined up volunteer help—not in a theoretical way, but in ink, on a calendar. Now that the babies have arrived, discourage unscheduled visits; if anyone says on the phone, "We'll stop in sometime next week," ask them not to do so unannounced. Instead, add their names to the calendar with times and *how each visitor plans to help in order to earn access.* As mentioned already, a worthwhile goal during the first month or two is to have someone, anyone, helping out at least a bit every day. If you still have any friends who haven't yet abandoned you due to your newly insufferable behavior, try to have them visit individually, not as a gaggle, and try to have at least one of them in per day to help out in whatever way she can.

After a few weeks of settling in to the rhythms of sharing jobs with legitimately hired help (like a baby nurse), stop and consider how well the arrangement is working for you. At the same time that you need to be reasonable and not ask too much of any one employee, you also need to be certain that you are using her efficiently and that she is providing genuine relief. If that is not the case, it is worth revisiting how you have parsed out jobs and whether or not that plan is effective. If you feel that the plan was a good one, but she's not honoring it, then sit down and talk to her unapologetically but diplomatically about your expectations. If you don't communicate clearly, the fault lies with you; she can't be expected to interpret your exasperated sighs with any specificity. The nanny market today is teeming, and you are likely to find someone who takes her work seriously—not as a fill-in between "real jobs," but as a career. Afford her the same benefits of clear communication of expectations and feedback on her performance that you would expect from your boss.

While it may seem at first that the job of organizing and delegating tasks is itself yet another burden, do not be fooled into thinking it would be easier just to do this all yourself. It may in fact be easier for a short while. Say, forty-five minutes.

The fact is that no one person could possibly perform all the duties associated with caring for twins and keeping a household intact. Remarkably, you will still have your hands full even with

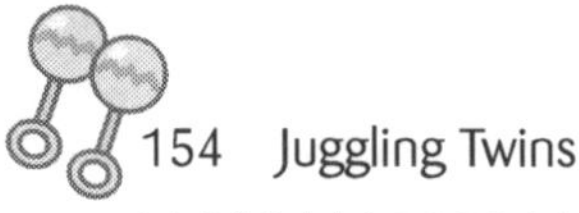



help. Hiring child care will change the character of your day from panicked hysteria to packed activity. This seemingly minor shift can be a disappointing discovery if you had imagined that hiring someone would lead to a charmed and queenly life for you. Your new life does in fact hold innumerable charms, two of whom will miraculously amplify their ability to charm you with every passing week. And yes, you are the queen. But this is a busy little kingdom you're ruling, and the work at the beginning is what it is—exhausting and abundant. Sharing the load with serfs remains far easier than cleaning the castle gutters yourself with two babies strapped to your chest.

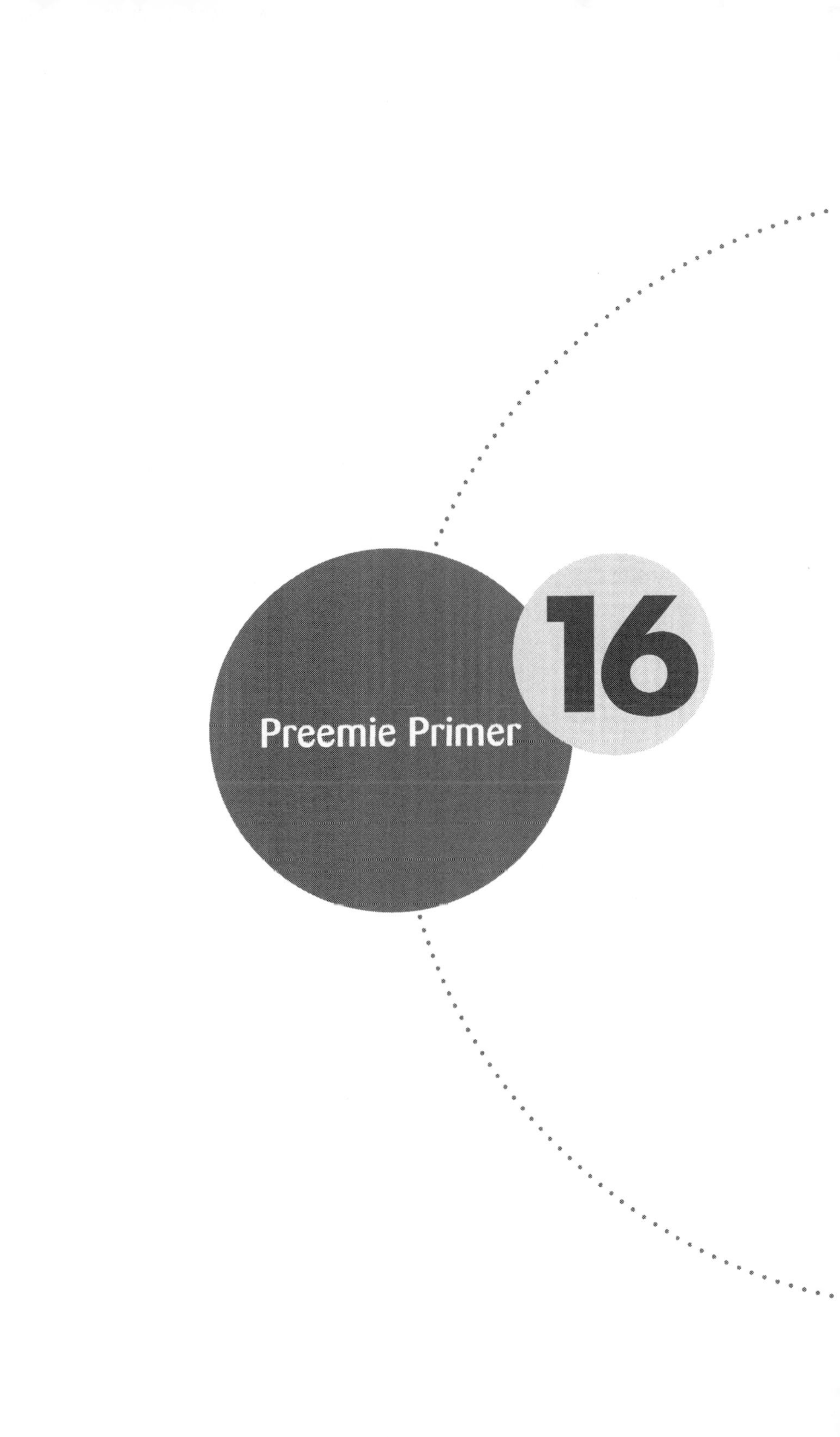
16
Preemie Primer

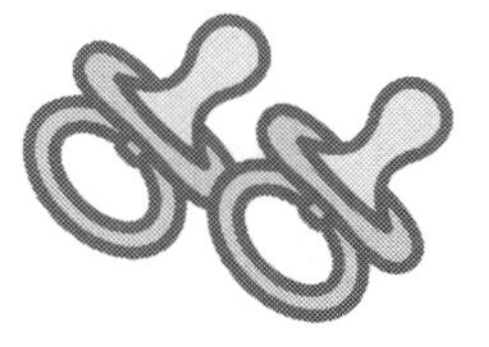

Premature births are on the rise in the United States, and it's important to educate yourself about this possibility since prematurity is far more likely with multiples. The rate at which babies have been born prematurely in the United States has increased nearly 30 percent in the last 25 years, and the number of us having twins has been one direct cause.[1] With twins, the rate of preterm birth tops 60 percent, and higher-order multiples are nearly always born prematurely.[2] The remarkable evolution that has occurred in neonatal care is also contributing to this dramatic increase in preterm birth rates. Twenty-eight weeks was once considered the threshold of probable survival for a premature baby, but today the mark is more realistically under 26 weeks. Recently, cases have been reported of babies surviving after entering the world at fewer than 22 weeks.

These increases mean that a tremendous number of families with twins are dealing not simply with the typical stresses of caring for two babies, but also with the challenge of raising two babies who have extraordinary needs. Excellent comprehensive resources are now available for the parents of the more than half a million preemies born every year, including medical and community websites, magazines, blogs, conferences, and even expos. Many hospitals do a good job of

---

1. March of Dimes Birth Defects Foundation, *Premature Birth Rate in U.S. Reaches Historic High* (March of Dimes, 2007).

2. National Center for Health Statistics, final natality data, http://www.marchofdimes.com/peristats (accessed November 19, 2007).

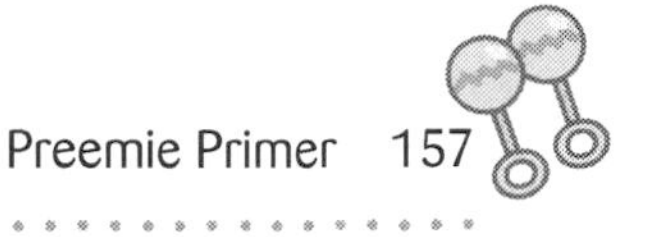

training new parents of preemies in the basics of providing special care before eventually sending them home after graduation from the NICU. At the same time, if your twins have been born prematurely, you need to be proactive about getting the information that you need to feel more confident about caring for them on your own. Use this time to gather all the information you can from the NICU nurses. They are not necessarily focused on educating you, but they can be a fantastic source of information, if you pursue them for it. Keep a notebook and pen with you to write down their answers to the many questions you have about how to care for your babies when they come home.

Here are a few essential pointers that will hopefully have been introduced to you by now but bear repeating. If you are new parents

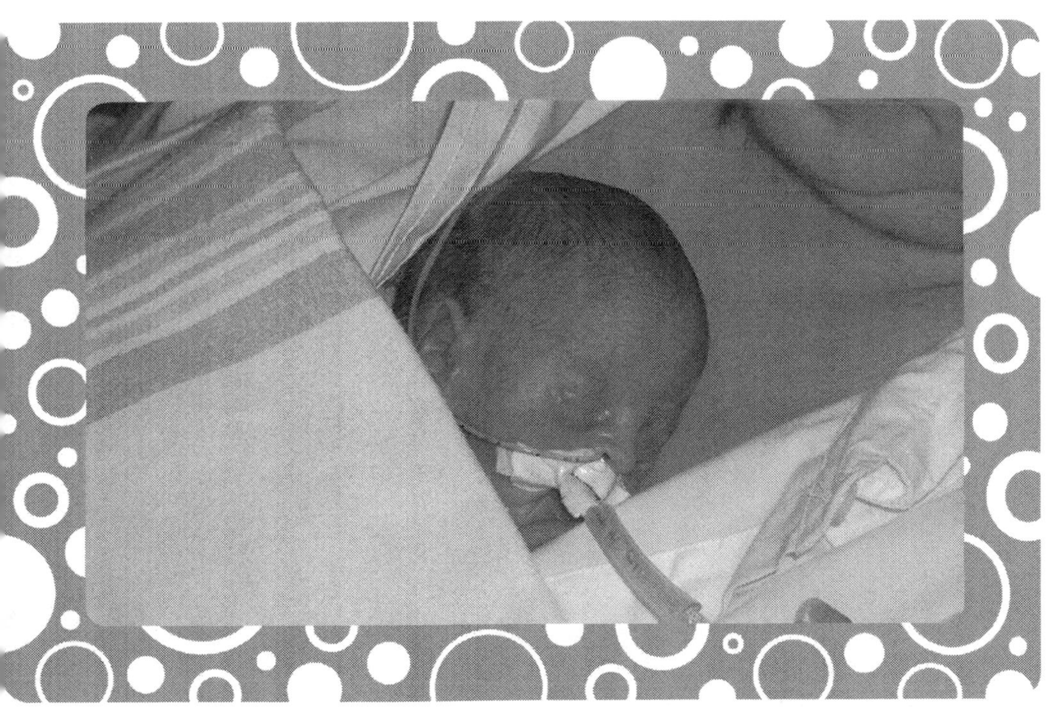

Each preemie twin needs plenty of skin-to-skin time with a parent.
Photo courtesy of Ruthbea and Neil Clarke

of preemies, these tips can serve as a primer as you begin to make your way through the complex web of resources now available for your education and support during this intense time.

## Tips for Parents of Preemie Twins

- Preemies in NICUs are often placed very close to each other when they sleep. Their proximity is considered important because the heartbeat of each baby stimulates and comforts the other. This is a bit trickier now that we know we need to place babies on their backs to sleep, but it can still be achieved if you swaddle each baby and then place them right next to each other, as closely situated as possible. Be sure to consult with your pediatrician about the safest and most medically helpful positions in which to sleep your babies.
- Give each baby as much time as possible lying skin-to-skin with you. A mom of preemies that I know says, "Bonding with babies in the NICU is very different from bonding with babies at home. You may not feel bonded, and this may cause feelings of guilt. Talk about this with the professionals in the NICU, or with your healthcare providers if the babies are home. Starting a scrapbook while the babies were in the NICU was very helpful for me. It helped me to look at their pictures when I was pumping at home, or just during times when I was away from one or both." Spending "skin time" with each baby is healthy for the babies and for you, too.
- Remember that your expectations about how your babies are developing need to be adjusted to their due date, rather than calculated from their birthday. If your twins were born eight weeks early, they will probably reach milestones at least eight weeks later than the books say babies will.
- When your babies are released from the NICU, either one at a

time or together, you will have an elaborate schedule of check-ups and check-ins for them—or perhaps orders to schedule these. In the midst of the craziness of beginning to take care of twin babies at home, remain very focused on getting to these appointments so that your babies' progress can be monitored carefully. Line up help for transportation, or if there are other children, schedule babysitting for them at appointment time.

- In addition to the information about intake and elimination, add to your daily chart a column for *temperature,* and monitor the babies' temps regularly. It is difficult for premature babies to stay warm and keep their temperatures up; it is also crucial that you know quickly if they are feverish, which could indicate that their immune systems are struggling to fight an infection.
- If you deliver prematurely, you should get a hospital-grade breast pump and begin pumping from day one. Your babies need the extra nutrition and immunity that your breast milk can provide, whether or not they are ready to latch on. If they can neither latch nor take a bottle, they will still be able to take your milk by tube in the NICU. In any case, get and meet with a lactation consultant while the babies are still in the hospital and then again when they are home. Some babies will need nipple shields to help them latch on, and a lactation specialist can help you use them and position the babies for breastfeeding.
- While it is tremendously challenging to deal with having one or both of your babies living in the NICU for an extended period, moms of preemies remind us that it is easier "in than out" of the hospital. Try to be patient.
- Try to find help with the babies in the form of only one or two hired hands or family members. The steady stream of infant-care volunteers suggested previously is *not* the right course of action for babies with compromised immune systems, though getting

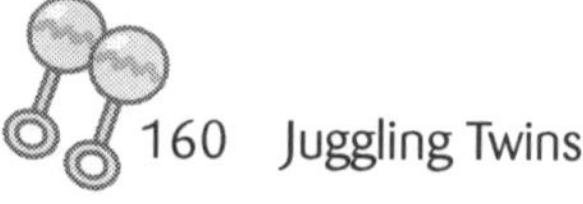


help with nonbaby duties will be critical. Postpone social baby visitations until a few weeks from now, minimally. Nobody with a cold comes near, and smokers need not even darken your doorstep. Stock up on hand sanitizer. Similarly, if your pediatrician doesn't allow you to wait in an exam room rather than in the virus-coated waiting room, get a new pediatrician.

- Before the babies are released from the NICU, alert your local fire department that you are bringing preemies home, so that your address is placed on a priority list and any calls made from your number are responded to immediately.
- Reconsider your work plans. You might need to take more time off from work than anticipated or give some thought to part-time options. Look into your eligibility for invoking the Family and Medical Leave Act in order to get invaluable time off for you or your partner.
- Resist comparing your twins to each other. This is perhaps even more important with preemies than it is with full-term babies and may be more tempting because you will be watching every ounce that you put in and every gain that each baby makes. Just as full-term infants will, preemies may respond to the same regimen differently and at their own pace.
- One important goal is to fatten these babies up. When you bottle-feed, be certain to heat the bottles carefully and consistently. The lower the temperature, the more calories the babies will use to consume and digest their meal. The idea is to increase their calories consumed and decrease calories expended to help them put on pounds.
- When supplementing with formula, choose one designed for density of calories. Generally, these add 22 calories to a bottle, which is a lot for someone that size. This is just as crucial if you are nursing, as your babies will need to eat very frequently, which

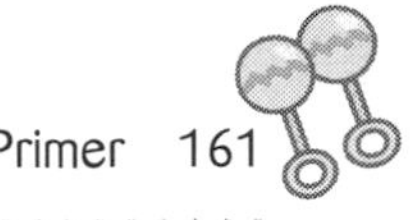

may exhaust you and your supply even more than the normal stresses of handling two infants. You want to get as much calorie-rich nutrition in these kids as you can; high-calorie formula can be a big help even if you are attempting to establish breastfeeding.

- Reflux is even more likely with premature babies. Do some quick research on preventing, recognizing, and handling reflux in newborns and be sure to mention it to your pediatrician if you suspect that one or both of your babies are exhibiting symptoms.

## Reach Out

And what about you? If we have already described the doubling of duties with twin babies as a scenario in which a mother is stretched to her limit, then what does this mean for a mother of twin preemies? In short, the added intensity of caring for the babies needs to be matched by an added intensity in your own care. You have not only been through labor—perhaps a sudden one—but have also probably weathered a host of exhausting emotions, including disappointment about the early birth, anxiety about the babies' outcome, and fear that their needs will overwhelm you. Moreover, you may have spent weeks or months traveling to and from the NICU, with some of those weeks possibly spent caring for one baby as you waited for the other to come home.

If you are to provide these babies the attention and care they need, you'll have to get good at accepting the attention *you* need, too. This is somewhere that friends and family can help. Be sure to remind your friends to call you every day, as this can be an incredibly isolating situation. While they may not yet be candidates for baby care, friends can certainly bring you meals, arrange playdates for your other children, sit with sleeping babies long enough to let you get a walk or a nap, or simply listen as you vent your mixed fear and elation at the birth of these tiny, precious babies. It is normal for you to have responses to this situation not unlike those associated with post-traumatic stress disorder; be on the lookout for signs of your own or your spouse's depression or anxiety, and seek appropriate treatment. You have no choice but to pay attention to your own needs if you are to effectively meet theirs. If raising twin babies can be likened to riding a roller coaster, then the ride for parents of preemie twins looks all the more daunting: the riders have boarded unwittingly, the hills are gargantuan, and the track is long. While the exhilarating highs may energize you to face the stomach-dropping lows, you still won't want to be riding alone. Reach out for help.

# 17

# Keeping Mom Healthy (and Sane)

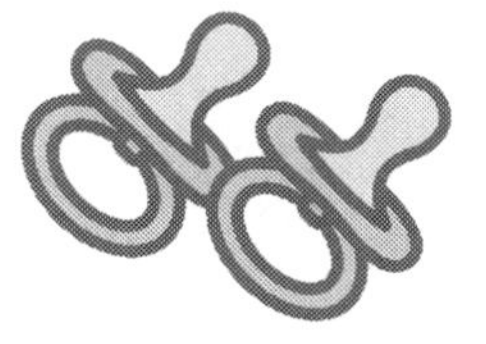

News flash: You no longer have the luxury of getting sick. Not only can you not stay in bed all day, but you no longer even have the option of harboring viruses. You must be an Immunity Superhero, fighting strep and the common cold with a consistent and steely determination, because (to maul the metaphor beyond recognition) this whole operation is a house of cards for which you are the base. Take that queen out of the bottom layer and the whole thing comes crashing down.

Your motherly instinct will kick in when it comes to protecting your kids from germy intrusions. Unless you are totally unschooled in the nature of viruses and their favorite vehicle—the uninvited children of friends and colleagues—by now you probably will have mounted a bottle of antiseptic squirt on each doorpost like little antibacterial mezuzahs. And you will discover soon enough that when a twin gets a cold, it's roughly fifteen or twenty minutes until the other comes down with it, which should serve to intensify your efforts to block the viral intrusion of your household. My children have never *not* shared an ailment other than splinters and tick bites.

But a misguided and illogical extension of your heroic efforts will be the regular abuse of your own body in a self-sacrificing endeavor to achieve martyrdom before the kids are in kindergarten. Obviously, you will not get enough sleep. Chances are you also won't eat well, particularly if you are no longer nursing or never did. The last time you will have sat down and relaxed on something other than a toilet or driver's seat is probably back when you needed help getting back out of your chair, and you may have decided that carrying 15-pound bundles up and down stairs all day is all the exercise you're really looking for, thank you very much. This just in from the Vatican: none of these forms of self-neglect qualify for sainthood anymore; they all went out with Vatican II.

## "When Mama Ain't Happy, Ain't Nobody Happy"

It may be easier for you to take care of yourself and stop hurling all your caretaking instincts in the solitary direction of your kids if you can believe in your gut that your health truly does affect the health of the family, and that you are now under some obligation to maintain it. Once you subscribe to this theory, you will feel freer to use some of your precious time to tend to your own basic health issues. You also need to convince your partner of the reasons you need to stay healthy. Your right to go for a walk, have a little time to yourself, and get enough sleep can't simply be occasional splurges. They are absolute, regular necessities. As one friend put it after she finally ended up on Prozac, having not carved out any time or attention for herself in ages, "When Mama ain't happy, ain't nobody happy." It is in the entire family's interest to support you on this. But you will have to take the lead.

Sanity is a good thing, and I'm all for it. The demands of caring for twins may be the first actual threat to your sanity that you've experienced, and may also lead you to the conclusion that what's really needed for your recovery to something resembling your formerly cheerful, resilient self is a couple of hours to hang out in a bookstore or go to a movie. These little treats seem like a great idea, but the awful truth is that breaks from the chaos are always too short, and the return to chaos two hours later can be rough once you've tasted some peace and quiet, especially if you return to a house that's in worse shape than you left it. At best, a field trip is a short-term fix. Even more important, I think, is to work on long-term, satisfying physical goals that can help you cope with the mental and emotional challenges. Once you've helped your body to be healthy, your mind will come along for the ride and will start feeling better, too.

At this early stage, you are still recovering from an arduous pregnancy and perhaps a tough delivery. Your body is keeping itself pretty busy just putting itself back together (think Scarecrow in *The Wizard of Oz*). It is remarkably good at this recovery process if you give it a fighting chance. That would seem like a reasonable proposition if you didn't have these babies to take care of, right? It is clichéd but true: in order to take care of them, you're going to have to take care of yourself, too. So what does that look like in the early days, when you hardly have time to empty your bladder?

## Sleep: Take It Whenever You Can Get it

Mostly, it comes down to grabbing sleep whenever there's a pocket of opportunity, be it a ten-minute power nap or a Sunday-morning sleep-in. This sounds obvious, but it is shockingly easy to squander spare moments that could be spent sleeping. Old habits die hard, including those created back when you actually had an occasional moment to yourself during which you weren't panting from exhaustion. The Internet is particularly good at tempting one from sleep time, and it has the further ability to warp time, as well; when you finally pull yourself away from that peek at an update on the personal lives of the stars of *Grey's Anatomy,* you may be surprised that the ten minutes you thought you had invested were actually forty. E-mail is similarly seductive, particularly because you have news to report and pictures to send to family and friends. While both of these are great ways to blow off steam, and the Internet can indeed be a great resource for you now, neither is truly as helpful as a nap. Dutifully report to bed whenever you are granted a reprieve.

Don't lose sight of the fact that you are still, at this point, a patient. In your first month home, you may be dealing with engorged breasts, constipation, recovery from surgery, soreness anywhere and everywhere from labor, the discomfort of episiotomy stitches or perineal tearing, and the cramping that happens as your uterus tries to find its way home. Even the combination of all of the above may not seem to you to be impressive, relative to the work of caring for these two babies. Still, you need to tend to these discomforts rather than shove your own recovery aside for the babies' sakes. The more quickly and completely you are up to speed, the more effectively you will be able to mother them. You're useless to them if you get good and sick because you have ignored your own body's messages. Just as we are instructed to adjust our own oxygen masks first in the unlikely event of cabin depressurization, you need now to grab that thing and breathe deeply before you can get on with the business of keeping the little people in your row alive.

# How to Get In and Out of Your Car and Other Things You Thought You Already Knew How to Do

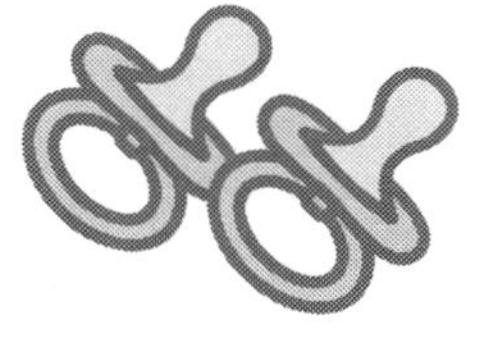

This is the issue that worried me most when I lay awake at night, and it tended to lead to others. I just couldn't picture it. Could I carry all my gear and two babies in infant seats out the back door, down four stairs, and out to the car in the driveway? What if I tripped? It can't be safe to carry two babies at once, right? But if I took just one baby out to the car, where would I leave the other one? And if I left the other one inside, then wouldn't I be leaving a baby in the car in order to come back in the house to get the one I left? And if you leave a baby in the car, don't they arrest you? And if they arrest me, will they at least get that baby out of the car and bring him in where it's warm before they take me away? And what about dinner that night? Who will make dinner that night if I'm in the slammer?

I didn't really come up with a theoretical solution; we just had to try it out once they arrived and we were ready to leave the nest. At first, it was simple. I never went out alone. I always had someone with me who could stay in the house with a baby to make sure the dog didn't snack on him while I took his brother to the car, or my assistant simply carried one out while I took the other. These early months are the easiest with this issue, actually, as the babies are still light and, most importantly, their wonderful car seats just pop in and out of the car with the babies happily fastened in them. You can spend as much time as you like getting them changed, dressed, situated, and snapped into their seats in the comfort of your kitchen, rather than wrestling with them in the back seat of the car. Going someplace in the car at this point is just a matter of getting the two seats into their bases.

However, once you are attempting to do this alone—which probably won't be in the first month unless you're foolhardy or you have one serious case of cabin fever—it gets a bit trickier. You will face a dilemma consisting of two apparently unsafe scenarios: leaving a child unsupervised momentarily or carrying two at once. I cannot, here in the Land o' Litigation, recommend either but can only tell you what I chose. Leaving one in the kitchen, strapped in a car seat, felt infinitely safer to me than descending stairs with a car seat in each hand. However, certain things had to be in place for me to get comfortable with this idea: I had to secure the dogs; I had to double check for anything within a ten foot area that could somehow land in the baby's mouth; I had to be certain that I didn't lock myself out of the house with the baby inside; and I had to sprint from the car back to the house once number one was in the car. Similarly, I couldn't leave the first baby in the car for those thirty seconds without other things in place: I had to warm the car but then turn it off and remove the key so that nobody could drive off with him; I had to double check that I had the seat locked properly in its base; and I had to make sure that I had not locked the keys in the car. An ordeal, to be sure. But it worked.

## Two Babies, One Set of Stairs

Some parents of twins have an even more complex situation to maneuver through, because they live in apartments with long flights of stairs to street level. My feeling is that unless there's a fire, there's never a good enough reason to carry two babies down stairs at the same time. Not in car seats, and certainly not out of them. There is only one good way to stop a fall if you begin to trip on the stairs, and that is to grab the rail, and there is only one way to grab the rail if your arms are full, and that is to toss your bundle. After thirty or forty years of stair climbing, you have developed by rote an instinct to grab that rail. And what will you toss? Well, "Down will come baaaaaaby…" Enough said. Imagining it should be a pretty good preventative.

I have heard of several solutions to this issue that mitigate the danger. One is to carry one baby on you in a cloth carrier. Then one baby gets carried in one arm, and the other hand is free to use the rail as you slowly descend. Some moms love the soft cloth baby carriers that put baby on their back as opposed to the Baby Bjorn types that carry them on the front, but I needed my back for the backpack/diaper bag that held my life in it. If this is your approach, though, the car seats stay in the car. This works well if you live in the city and your parking spot is God Knows Where, but it requires that the stroller is already in the car and that you don't forget one thing in the apartment, as you're certainly not leaving the babies down the street or double parked in front of the building in order to go up and retrieve a stroller or your forgotten cell phone.

Other solutions I've heard include putting them in a side-by-side stroller and ever so slowly backing it down the stairs, one stair at a time. This would scare me with visions of the three of us catapulting backwards, but I know it has been done without incident. My absolutely favorite solution, because it truly epitomizes the occasional ridiculousness of having two babies at once, is to sit down on the top stair with a baby in each arm and then scootch down the stairs on your butt, one at a time. I'm guessing this works better in pants than a skirt. I admit to doing this myself inside the house, simply trying to get us all from the second floor to the first. I salute the brave women who have done this in public, and I look forward to the day when I see a mother of twins doing this at Macy's because the escalator has stopped.

Once the babies can hold their heads up and therefore can ride in a backpack with a frame, usually at five or six months, carrying one in the pack and one on your hip—again with that free hand clutching the rail—becomes another option. Carrying them at that stage is harder in that they are heavier, but easier in that they are less wobbly. You'll be as strong as a bull by then from months of carrying them, so the weight won't even faze you. A dear friend recalls doing the dishes every night with one baby strapped on his back and the other on his front. His twins are now in college and canoed over one thousand miles across the Arctic wilderness with him last summer, carrying all their collective gear on long portages around waterfalls. What goes around comes around.

## Other Snares, Traps, and Mazes

### Locking Yourself In; Locking Yourself Out

The only way to prevent this scenario, which actually isn't very far-fetched at all, is to have a spare set of two keys—one for the house and one for the car—in your pocket at all times when you go out. Do not put it in your diaper bag or purse; you will absolutely lock the bag wherever you have locked the other key and baby. Do not put it under a rock in the backyard; this will not help you in the parking lot at the pediatrician's office as your two babies smile at you angelically from their car seats and you stand outside pawing wildly at the door handles in disbelief. Carry that spare set of keys on you until the kids are old enough to be able to unhook their car seats and open a car door for you (at least three and a half). If that sounds a little over the top, stop and think about the times you have locked yourself out of either place in the last five years and add a baby or two to the scene. Right. Spare set, in the pocket. Don't worry that the keys will *ruin the line* of your outfit. You no longer have a line. (See "Life in the Fat Lane.")

At the door that you usually use to exit with the babies, tape the following list, with your own additions, at eye level. Before leaving, be sure you have each item so that you don't need to return to the house once you are all safely strapped into the car. Our list also included a few chores like clearing all pacifiers and baby toys that a dog might devour if left out, as well as turning off lights and turning down the heat, as all of this preservation of twins is moot if they have no planet to live on. For us, anything we carried was pretty much all loaded into our diaper backpack, which also served as a purse.

## Exit-Door Check-Off List

- ☐ Spare keys
- ☐ Minimum of 10 diapers
- ☐ Wipes
- ☐ Changing pad
- ☐ Ointment
- ☐ Pacifiers
- ☐ Three full changes of clothes
- ☐ Prepared bottles, on ice packs
- ☐ Cell phone, charged
- ☐ Wallet

## Bathing Two

If you have never bathed an infant before, you're in for a nerve-racking but wonderful experience. The first time you hold a slippery infant in a tub, you will produce enough adrenaline to lift a car. (Do not attempt this until after the bath.) It is *scary* to have your little one wriggling around—possibly unhappily—in water, near the hard surface of a tub. It requires your full attention and both hands, which is why you certainly can't bathe two babies at once; you really shouldn't even try to bathe one baby while the other is in your care, in case the non-bather has issues of her own. Whereas you will soon

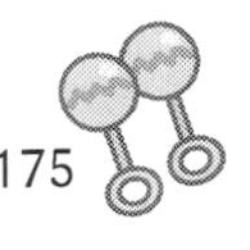

get pretty good at doubling up on some tasks, like feeding them, you won't be able to bathe them together safely until they can sit up reliably, which isn't for months. Until then, think of bath time as alone time with each of them. That's a good thing. They need it, and so do you. And bath time is a great opportunity to play, nuzzle, and bond with a baby.

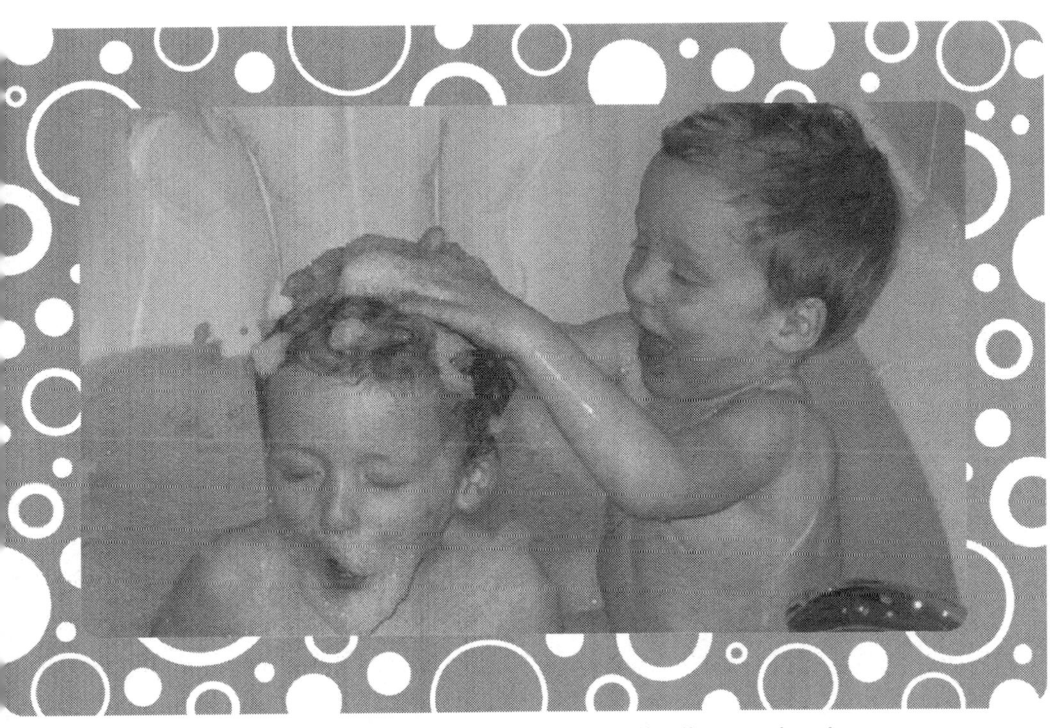

It will be a while before your twins are this self-sufficient in the tub.

Photo courtesy of the Regan-Loomis family

That said, you don't need to bathe a newborn every day unless you want to create that bonding time or incorporate bathing as part of a bedtime routine. Young babies don't really get dirty. We only bathed ours a couple of times a week at the beginning, and they were no less popular with their peers as a result. Babies don't get B.O.; they are designed to smell heavenly. Until they spit up, that is. Major spit up is indicative of its being a bath day. In general, though, don't stress about not fitting a bath in every day for each of them. It is totally reasonable at the beginning to alternate bath days between the babies. Try to limit this practice to the babies, however. You and your partner should in fact make a decent attempt to maintain your previous commitment to bathing even when you have not spit up on yourselves. Chances are pretty good that someone else has, anyway.

## Venturing Outside the House

Once you have actually left the house, you may find that the outing itself is less stressful than the exit scene. While it is true that my twins pretty much screamed every minute they were riding in the car for the first few weeks, there came a moment in the third week of delivering their sister to day camp when she said to me, "Hey, Mom. I can hear you!" because, for the first time, they were not simultaneously screeching. Once they got the knack, they seemed to enjoy the ride and would often fall asleep in the car. After that point, I ventured out to stores with them to pick up a few groceries or return all those 0–3-month clothing gifts that we would never get them into. It was healthy on so many levels to be out, and it was good training for the coming years to begin building up a reserve of snappy replies to the blinking, quasi-idiotic question that would assault us on virtually every outing for the first few years: "Oh! Twins?" Here are a few possibilities for you to put in your Retort Bank:

- "No. One of them is mine, but I found the other one out in the parking lot. Is it yours?"
- "Nope. They're clones, actually. We have six more at home just like them."
- "What are you talking about? Do you see two?"

## Two Babies, One Hullabaloo

One scene will repeat itself relentlessly during your first few months with these darlings, and it can be unnerving. When two babies cry desperately and simultaneously, even the steeliest of us get rattled. There's a good chance this will happen to you many times...in a given day. Here's the plan, when it happens:

1. Stay calm. You can get them both happy, and you don't have to do it in under two minutes. Breathe. Approach them not in a panic but with composure.
2. Assess the situation, and then do the *unobvious*. See who is crying most loudly and then tend to the *other* one. Here's my theory: if you have two babies crying, one at seventy decibels and one maxing out at about ninety-five, you should deal with the seventy first, before it too becomes ninety-five. That way, you have a cumulative total of 165, whereas if you tend to Mr. Squeaky Wheel first, his cohort will be at a full ninety-five by the time you have him calm, and then you'll have a total of 190. More simply: if you walk into a room in which you find one baby fully upset and one half upset, deal with the half before it too becomes a whole. The fully upset one *can't get any more upset* and might in fact get bored or fall asleep (don't count on it). But there's still room for escalation with the half-upset baby. Stem it.
3. Yes, if you are alone, one of the babies will have to continue to cry as you comfort the other. The baby will not, however, spontaneously combust. Neither will he or she begin hatching theories about your substandard parenting or obvious favoritism of the other. It is not a full-out disaster for a baby to cry for a while. You will get there. All will be well. Everybody relax. That means you, too.
4. Try not to cry yourself. That really confuses things. Wait until they stop, then take your turn, if necessary.

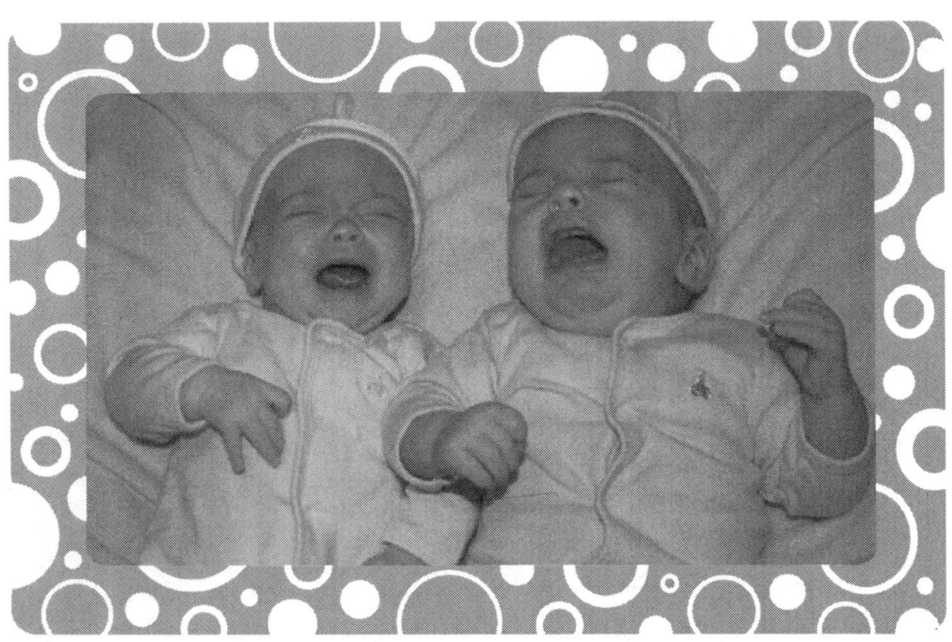

This, too, shall pass.

Photo courtesy of Kim and Stephen Brown

## Remember to Lighten Up

While the extraordinary blessing of twins demands a certain reverence—a deep-in-the-gut awe for this glorious miracle—it also requires a firm irreverence if you are to survive your own miracle. Your ultimate challenge is not how to feed these kids or get them in their car seats or fight your own fatigue; actually, the heart of the whole operation is maintaining your sense of humor. If you don't lighten up at times, if you don't look at each other and laugh as both babies are screaming and the smell of your own soured, spit-up breast milk curls up to your nostrils from your own shoulder, if you don't shrug those milk-soured shoulders and shake your head and laugh from the bottom of your belly, then I'm afraid you are lost.

Unless you chortle at this insanity regularly and forgive your spouse all perceived baby blunders daily, just as you are forgiven your bossiness and hormonal outbursts, then you, my friend, are sunk. Because something will have to give. It might be some portion of your sanity. It might be your marriage. But without a valve, this finely tuned stress machine will surely blow.

The perfect-parent-perfect-baby intentions we brought to the raising of our eldest might have gone out the window with our second child even had he not been born simultaneously to our third. Surely we all fall into that parent trap a bit with first children and can laugh at ourselves a bit more with subsequent siblings. The difference with subsequent *twins* seems to be how *far* those intentions get flung out the window. Ours made it to the next town.

Calibrating your expectations is in fact a crucial survival maneuver. *Lower that bar!* Flout your own standards and devise a new checklist for parenting that doesn't include the babies' regular exposure to classical music and color wheels designed to stimulate the visual cortex, daily motor-skill-development exercise routines, or carefully chosen organic food for the entire family, prepared beautifully and presented lovingly. At the end of the day, try this checklist, instead:

- ☐ Is everyone still alive?
- ☐ Has anyone wandered off, or are we all still accounted for?
- ☐ Has everyone bathed this month? (Okay, has *any*one?)
- ☐ Did food pass over everybody's lips at some point today?
- ☐ Has anyone seen or heard from the dog today?
- ☐ Are there any clean(ish) clothes ready for tomorrow?

*continued...*

- ☐ Are we up-to-date on paying bills to the point that we will have heat and electricity again tomorrow?
- ☐ Have we laughed today?
- ☐ No, seriously, guys. Where's the dog?

Here's a revelation that shouldn't be earth-shattering to you by now: *this is really hard*. Having two babies at once is *really, really* hard. And in the first month, you are in the thick of it—the hardest part of hard. Great, wonderful, amazing, inspiring, and lucky...but hard, hard, *hard*. So, guess what? If you feel tired, overwhelmed, and at times utterly incompetent, you're right on course. It is a laudable accomplishment just to keep it together and to keep everyone healthy at the beginning.

When James Taylor wrote the line, "Holdin' it together ain't always easy," little could he predict the relevance it would have when he eventually became a 53-year-old father of twins. You could simply sing that line to yourself for a few months as a soothing reminder of your not being alone in the chaotic world of twin parenting. We actually adopted the chant that Eddie Murphy's character in the sleeper classic *Bowfinger* soothes himself with when under duress: "keep-it-together-keep-it-together-keep-it-together..." It helped. We coped. You will, too.

# Part III
# Weeks Four to Twelve

Did you spend any time at all in an arcade when you were a kid? If so, you remember the Whac-a-Mole. For a quarter, you could take a mallet and try to smash the heads of little furry (fake) moles that popped up and then quickly receded into five little holes on the tabletop. (It was recently revitalized by the great TV commercial featuring Venus Williams knocking her first mole senseless—so hard that the others refused to surface.) For the next couple of months, and to some degree for the next several years, this is your life. Just as you think you have quelled all the demands of your day, just as you have knocked off four tasks at once and can sit back on your heels for half a second, just as that mole table looks cleared...*Pop!* goes the weasel. In order to cope with your constant to-do list—the chores, thank-you cards, grocery runs, appointments and, oh yeah, the babies—you will need to revert to your twelve-year-old Whac-a-Mole sensibility.

When you played that game, you never entertained fantasies about the moles relenting. You knew they would return. In fact, you waited with intense anticipation for that next little smashable mole noggin. It is time to tap back into that mindset. The demands of your new life will pop at you with that same velocity and that same menacing insinuation of mockery that those cheerful little moles had. You just have to keep swinging, knowing you can't fully clear the table. You have to return to your Whac-a-Mole days. You have to go *back* to the *whac*.

# 19 Sleeping and Eating: Holdin' It Together Still Ain't Easy

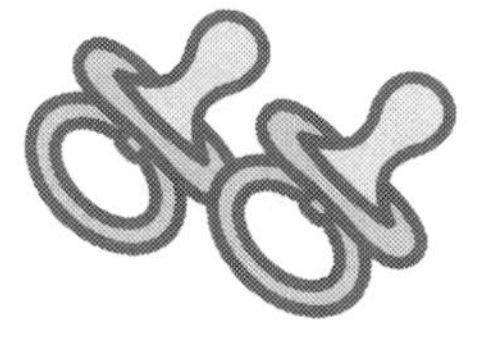

For various reasons, this stage is just plain difficult. While you are working determinedly to get your twins to comply with a schedule, they're probably not there yet; there are still plenty of nights that are wild free-for-alls, and there are plenty of days when those six or seven feedings for each baby somehow seem to turn into eleven...and they are *still* cranky. You are moving from the relatively chaotic first month to a period of established routines that is not yet set, and the intervening period can be rocky and frustrating. The continued effort to slide everyone onto that same page of sleeping and eating on a schedule becomes so important, and it takes perseverance to try day after day when the message doesn't seem to be getting through to the two central participants in the program.

## Reality Check

When our babies were three months old, I met a woman at a party who as a single mom had raised twin girls who were heading off to college that week. She shook her head as she looked at our boys and said, "When my girls were that age, every night around sunset, I would start crying. The nights were pure torture." Her memory of the period was still unduly vivid, and perhaps with good reason.

The feeding program remains the same as it was presented in the section on month one, adjusted of course for the babies' weights, their increasing intake, and their expanding ability to wait longer between feedings. The difference now is that slowly, slowly, as they get bigger and become more comfortable in their world, they will begin to fall into step with the program that you have been lovingly suggesting to them all along. The issue of sleep is particularly challenging now, though. Babies at this age are too young to sleep train ("cry it out") but are still prone to feeling unsettled and overstimulated. The daily effort to produce meaningful sleep periods in scheduled chunks may fall flat repeatedly. But still, *keep trying.*

At twelve pounds, most babies can string together four to six hours of sleep. That twelve-pound benchmark generally happens somewhere in this two-to-four-month range, but sometimes even later. You're getting your hopes up now, aren't you? You're looking at your eleven-and-a-half pound babies and imagining that you'll be sleeping six straight hours tonight, starting at midnight? Sorry, but the first time they do it, it will probably be between 7:30 p.m. and 1:30 a.m., and then they will wake up and wonder where the party is. And unfortunately, babies are notoriously bad planners and less-than-perfect communicators (yes, even with each other, in spite of all that stuff you've been reading about twin telepathy). They will seldom coordinate their plans so that these initial longer stretches happen simultaneously. Instead, the scenario will likely look something like this:

## A Typical Scenario

1. Baby A falls asleep at 9:45 p.m., Baby B at 10:28 p.m. Both of them down, you enjoy a blissful moment of peace and furtively think, *Okay! This isn't so bad!* A little giddy with the quiet, you neglect to go straight to bed and instead trundle over to the computer to read e-mails from four days ago. *Just fifteen minutes,* you tell yourself.

2. At 12:45 a.m., foggy eyed before the computer screen, you are rattled from your trance by a cry. You breathe deeply and trudge to the nursery, where Baby A is suggesting in her special, piercing way that feeding her immediately would be the recommended course of action. To your surprise, Baby B sleeps on.

3. At 1:30 a.m., just finishing feeding Baby A, you wait anxiously for the second cry from the nursery, but it doesn't come. In a brief, dark flash, it occurs to you that Baby B has in fact perished, but you are at once afraid to check and unwilling to risk waking him up if it turns out that he has not. You chase the thought away and focus on Baby A's gas.

4. At 2:10 a.m., you are having some difficulty convincing Baby A, now fed, changed, and re-swaddled, that it would be prudent to go back to sleep. You rock, cajole, bounce, swaddle, re-swaddle, re-rock, and walk her until, at 2:50 a.m., she finally passes out and you are able to put her down and head to bed. On your way out, you pause by Baby B's crib and are assured by the sound of his tiny grunting and wheezing that he has not in fact perished. Relieved beyond reason and delighted that he is sleeping so long, you stumble to bed. Job well done. You're beat. It is now 3:00 a.m. and you fall into sleep as if falling from a cliff, into a deep, black crevice, falling, falling heavily toward nirvana…

5. At 3:28 a.m., Baby B, having just slept for five hours straight for the first time, awakens famished and furious. "Wha—?" you stammer, crawling back up the cliff wall to consciousness. You lug yourself to the nursery to begin another feeding. Rather than celebrating Baby B's major milestone, you begin whimpering uncontrollably.

If you have been paying attention, you'll know that the biggest problem with this picture happens in Step 1. You're not even supposed to be awake at that time of night! A reminder concerning your own sleep training: *You need to go to bed after the feeding that precedes the 10 p.m. feeding, be it at 7:30 p.m. or 9 p.m.* If you do so, and someone else takes charge of the 10 p.m. top-off, then you are free to sleep until the babies wake up, which in any scenario is likely to be sometime after 1 a.m. No matter what happens the rest of the night—whether they stay up and party or decide tonight's the night to sleep through—you will at least have five or six hours of sleep under your belt. And if you think you'll never be able to get to sleep at 7:30 p.m., well…yes, you will.

## Tactics for Encouraging Longer Stretches of Sleep

The biggest challenge of the period between four weeks and twenty is that the babies can neither be fully sleep trained (yet) nor relied upon to adhere to the schedule you are creating for them. Still, you try, and the most immediate goal in the process is to make it possible for them to put together that four-to-six-hour stretch of sleep. A number of tactics can help:

- If you haven't yet established the bedtime routine discussed in "Coping with the Nights" (page 129), now is the time. Whatever regimen you decide upon, be religious about it. Sleep training, even in these preliminary stages, is all about consistency.
- Once you are trying for longer stretches, your babies should be sleeping in cribs, not in bouncy seats or car seats.
- Put the babies down to bed *earlier* in order to get more sleep out of them. It's totally counterintuitive, but it works. We put our guys down by 6:30 p.m. at the latest, which is the time that most sleep-training books recommend. Yes, it may mean the worker bee in the family doesn't get to see the babies in the evening. Don't fret; chances are, there will be plenty of time to visit in the middle of the night.

- Try to make the 10 p.m. feeding a "dream feed" by entering their room in the dark, totally silently, and slipping them the bottle or the breast.
- Begin reducing the amount of formula you give during later night feedings. Some moms promise that without the incentive of a big bottle, babies won't bother waking. Others even water down the formula or give a "mini-bottle" rather than a full one in the middle of the night. There is also a contingent that puts rice cereal in the 10 p.m. feeding in order to keep the babies fuller longer. (If you do so, wait until they are at least fifteen pounds, and then get bottles with X or Y nipples or cut a regular nipple with an X-Acto knife so that the rice/milk cocktail can get through the hole.) None of these was our approach, but others swear by them.
- If nursing, note that you are at your most diminished supply of breast milk for the day just when they need a big bellyful—at that 10 p.m. feeding. Consider introducing a bottle of formula in order to tank them up at that last feeding. We did this, and it definitely helped. The premixed formulas are heavier than the powdered and are a better choice for this feeding.
- Before automatically feeding them at every wake-up call, try a few minutes of soothing them back to sleep. Visitations between 10 p.m. and 6 a.m. should be strictly business. Re-swaddle an unwrapped baby, rub her belly, leave a hand on her until she's asleep and then try to safely remove it, perhaps finger by finger. But don't inspire the babies to wake up at this hour by making these sessions sweet bonding times. Get in and get out. Change them only if absolutely necessary (consider double diapering or adding a sanitary pad to each diaper to get them through without a change). Once they are through the night, after all, you won't be waking them to change their diapers.
- Moderate pressure on your baby—a hand on her belly—can make

her feel more secure and might work in lieu of picking her up to rock her and then you won't have to face the whole getting-her-back-down-asleep predicament.

- If the babies still seem to calm when swaddled but are starting to get out of the swaddle while sleeping, double up. Put them in onesies so that there's no chance of overheating, then swaddle them twice, each time tightly. This technique bought us a couple of extra months of swaddling. Remember if you double swaddle to use breathable cotton blankets so that the babies don't overheat.
- Adjust the daily schedule by adding a bottle (or a few ounces per bottle) during the day to anticipate one fewer bottle at night.
- If the babies share a room and you suspect that one is starting to wake the other with crying, set up a Pack-n-Play in your room for the troublemaker—or better yet, move the whole crib—until the situation improves.
- Toward the three-month mark, gradually stop waking the second baby for a feeding if you have fed the other. This may be a rough transition, but it is crucial if they are to start sleeping through the night.

Most of us hear the news that babies *might* sleep longer at twelve pounds the way we need to hear it—that they *will* do so. Then, when their babies don't oblige, moms think something is wrong with their babies. Potential does not equal performance, however. Your babies may or may not be ready to sleep longer at that time. While it's likely that this is just a developmental issue, there may be other factors that are keeping them from doing so, and they may be issues that give them difficulty during the daylight hours as well. Gas may be the culprit, as it can really make a baby uncomfortable. Teething is possible, too. These are standard suspects. One that is less known but can really give a baby a hard time is reflux.

## Reflux in Babies

Technically, all babies have some measure of reflux, since it involves the underdevelopment of a valve between the esophagus and the stomach that keeps swallowed food where it belongs, and babies are born without its being totally developed. It's the reason babies spit up a lot. The valve tends to be fully functioning by six months, but in the meantime, many babies really struggle with the symptoms the situation produces. Be on the lookout for back arching, funny faces (when a baby tastes acids), a white mouth (again, stomach acid), discomfort when laid flat, and lots of spitting up.[1] Many cases of reflux have likely been deemed "colic" over the years. As an immediate help, remember to sleep your babies on an incline, either by propping the crib or sleeping them in bouncy seats or car seats. If you truly suspect that one or both of your babies has reflux, get an appointment with the pediatrician or a pediatric GI, who may prescribe an appropriate dosage of Zantac or, if that doesn't help, Prilosec.

Perhaps this is obvious, but you should not play Dr. Mom and decide without consulting a doctor that your babies would benefit from trying these drugs. This is also true of teething remedies and even Tylenol, ibuprofen, and cough and cold medicines. I find it astonishing to see parents online advising other parents to try Tylenol if the baby seems cranky, because "it could be teething," or to "give Zantac a shot in case it's reflux." Criminal! These are tiny, ten-pound bodies we're talking about, and powerful drugs that affect these bodies *dramatically*. Very casually, one mom on a message board that I read recommended to another that she try Benadryl to help her wakeful baby sleep through the night. I wanted to call the police! Not only is medicating a child through a normal developmental stage totally unethical (and clearly more for the benefit of the parent than the child), but that drug isn't even designed as a sleep aid. Sleepiness is a possible *side effect*. (So is wakefulness, by the way.)

1. "Silent reflux" involves all but the spitting up.

If you look at the directions, you'll see that the FDA doesn't even approve dosage amounts for ages 0–2 for most of these products. In a word, don't try to mask or medicate the characteristics of infancy away, especially if you don't even have a diagnosis.

## Pacifiers

For the majority of this stage, the swaddle and the pacifier are your new best friends. Toward the end of it, though, you may find one or both of your babies beginning to Houdini out of the swaddle, and you will also recall that it's getting to be time to jettison the binkie. As for the swaddle, our boys would have gladly stayed in theirs until the summer before leaving for college. At three years old, they still like to be wrapped up tightly in blankets when they look at books. Some babies get squirmy, though. Before you simply give up on the swaddle and loose their limbs on the world, try swaddling with one arm out. This way, they are able to get a thumb or whole hand to their mouths to suck.

As for the pacifier, just bear in mind that it's much easier to eliminate at three months than it is at six, and it's incalculably easier now than it is when they are old enough to shout, "Give me binkie!" while throwing themselves at your feet. We were fortunate in that our kids showed no visible reaction to this deprivation, which we pulled off right at three months. If yours do resist, you'll have to resort to an intervention.

### The Four-Step Program for Pacifier Detox

1. Aim to rid the household of all binkies by the time the children are three months old. Do not exceed four months. With every week that passes, the process will become more painful for the addicts. This includes you.

*continued...*

2. Start by putting the pacifiers away during the day, then work on the nights. Try two days *sans binque,* then toss those little suckers, as it were.
3. Before you throw them away, cut the tops off, rendering them useless. Parents have been known on night two to dig through the trash—not the trash in the house, but the trash cans out by the garage—in desperation to find them. There is a *reason* that drug addicts flush their pills down the toilet rather than throw them in a wastebasket. Do not flush the pacifiers down the toilet, however. They might float back to the top in the middle of the night, and you will be tempted to pluck them out.
4. Plan to have three really crummy nights. Don't turn back. Use every other method of comforting that has ever worked for your kids, including letting them suck on your appendages.

Again, this is the trickiest stage where sleep is concerned. Gone are the days when the babies could be plopped down asleep and counted on to stay asleep even as you vacuumed the cobwebs over their cribs. Instead, you are learning to walk with a sleeping baby as softly as a Sioux squaw in her moccasins from the rocker to the crib, to place him in the crib, to stand there bent over the rail with your hands stuck under him, and then, over the course of, say, seven minutes, to slide your hands from under him so gradually that your movements are imperceptible to the human eye. This is trickier still if, like me, you are not 23 years old. Standing up straight after marathons like that, my back would crunch so loudly that I'd wake the baby anyway. In any case, these are the weeks to gut out. A few months down the road, these sleep challenges will be ironed out (mostly), and it will begin to seem plausible that you, too, will be able to get more than three hours of sleep at a time. In the meantime, you are not alone. Somewhere across town, other parents of twins are awake with you at 3:41 a.m. Hang in there.

# 20

# Time to Get Out of the House

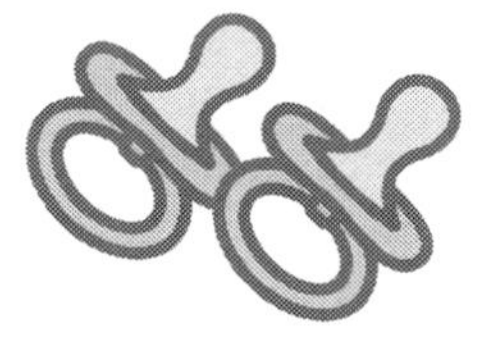

It's easier to stay home.

Don't.

Whether you were already a stay-at-home mom caring for the twins' older sibling(s) or you are taking a break from a career, if you are staying home as the primary caretaker of your babies, you now face a host of new challenges in your life. Not the least of these is occasionally feeling like a caged animal. I've heard full-time baby care described as "mind-numbing" and devoid of "mental stimulation." I disagree entirely. There is so much to learn, so much that is foreign, and so much that is truly fascinating about newborns in general and twins in particular. Besides, since when has being in love with two people at once ever not been an interesting challenge? I can't say I ever felt bored, exactly, being home with my guys. At the same time, there are few jobs outside the home, other than that of soldier or lighthouse keeper, that require that you never leave the workplace—that you eat and sleep onsite, operate in isolation, move mostly between just a few rooms and, oh yes, clean them as you work. Even if you love your home, you're going to find yourself knocking your head against one of its walls repeatedly if you don't occasionally leave it for some fresh air.

During the first month, you may forget that another world even exists outside your baby bunker. Perfectly understandable. As you move through the second and third months, however, you may at some point catch a glimpse of the world beyond your windows and realize that the last outing you took was when you ran that errand to the labor and delivery room a while back. Beginning to lay the foundation of a schedule and a routine, you now move from the immediate hubbub of excitement, visitors, and a triage sensibility to a more stable day, a plan, and perhaps a growing independence as the world ebbs back into itself and leaves you to tend to these babies. That's good and bad. You are likely experiencing an emerging sense of confidence that you can do this, even on your own, and perhaps even an interest in reclaiming your space and time from visitors, as helpful as they have been. As this happens, however, you may also sometimes miss the attention and the adult interaction. You may in fact feel isolated.

## Danger Zones

A number of in-home temptations exist that can seem to take the edge off your seclusion while potentially exaggerating the problem. Television and the Internet are special danger zones. TV is alluring perhaps because there are other adults on it and, like the cat who looks longingly at television images of birds and mice, you are looking hungrily at images of other full-grown humans on the *Today* show. Be selective and disciplined. It might make sense to allow yourself a morning show or a recorded episode of *Desperate Housewives* (because you're not allowed to stay up late enough to watch new episodes, of course), but then you must turn the thing off. Don't leave it on for background companionship. In the first place, it's bad for the babies.[1] Secondly, you may unwittingly get drawn in to shows that are truly just mind-numbing time sucks. Use TV sparingly and judiciously, just as you will have your children do once they are old enough.

1. American Academy of Pediatrics, Committee on Public Education, *Children, Adolescents, and Television,* policy statement, February 2001, *Pediatrics* 107:423–6.

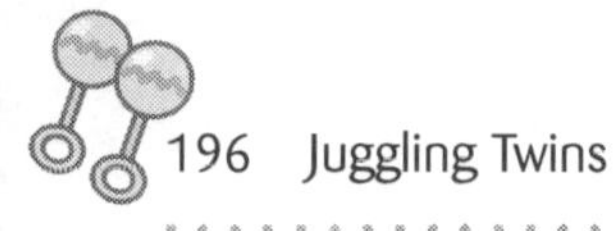


If you really need some auditory companionship, listen to music. While the Mozart Effect has been mostly debunked[2] and your children are no longer guaranteed admission to Yale simply because they listened to *Eine kleine Nachtmusik* in the womb, there is no doubt that music calms the savage beast, and that includes beastly infants. Having good music playing in the house will help all three of you get through the day and is in the end a better companion for you than the tortured protagonist of an afternoon soap.

The Internet is tricky, though. Some days, it may be your lifeline. I became an addict of my online Mothers of Twins group—comprised of others who had twins in my area and were asking and getting answers to shared questions—and this was mostly a productive use of time. But random searching on baby questions or any medical concerns can be misleading and can direct one so quickly to alarmist arguments based on dubious research—the shoddiness of which is difficult to detect for a nonmedical, casual reader. Pediatricians spend a lot of time divesting parents of anxieties produced by over-the-top Internet sites. At the same time, the Internet can be an amazing resource for parents, and there are so many great troves of information out there (see Resources section) that may in fact help to relieve worries you have about your children's health or behavior. The bottom line is probably that sleep—yours—comes first when you have both babies settled, and the Internet a distant second.

As you settle in to a routine, you may be ready to pursue some small take-home work projects or even a few minutes of reading or a hobby now and then, when both babies are sleeping. This is the beginning of reclaiming yourself, and it's important to take this step. If it requires your brain in the least, you might want to consider doing it for a few minutes during the babies' morning nap, as your cognitive functioning is not guaranteed later in the day. Leave the

---

2. Alison Abbott, "Mozart Doesn't Make You Clever," *Nature.com,* April 2007 (accessed November 20, 2007).

floor unswept and the egg-coated plates coagulating in the kitchen sink in order to read for the twenty minutes you are granted when they are both asleep. Eventually, you'll get the dishes done somehow, but you may not get another twenty minutes to yourself that day, or they may come when you're running on cerebral fumes. Just sit down in the middle of the mess and read or work on a document or start that baby journal. Whatever makes you feel human.

There is a certain irony in the possibility that after you work for months to create a routine, you may begin shortly thereafter to hate its regularity. Every regimen needs its breaks. I found this need swelling when the kids were three months old and we were starting to come up for air. Before that, I hardly remembered that I existed as an individual, let alone one who needed time off now and then. A fish doesn't know she's in water.

## Goals for Mom

Those of us who are making the transition from a workplace are often accustomed to a goal-driven structure, and it might help to bring that practice home. In addition to the goals of keeping the babies fed, warm, and happy, you can set goals regarding your own continued sanity. For example, it would be reasonable to have the following as goals:

- getting out at least twice per week with the twins;
- getting out once per week alone; and
- having a date night (yes, without your kids) at least once a month.

If you are of the truly goal-driven ilk, you also may want to think about having a target or purpose to your every day at home—to introduce something new to the babies, to finish three thank-you

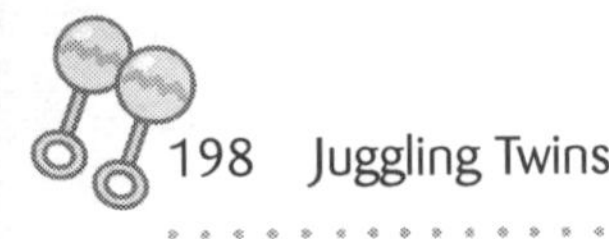


cards, to cook dinner rather than order in—whatever it takes to give you a more specific objective than the over-arching, fundamental goal of keeping the family intact. Whether or not you are one of these go-getter girls, you will realize at some point that in order to remain active in adult society, you will need to go to it. It will not keep coming to you, even though it threatened to do so when the kids were first born. You'll need to be proactive about getting out of your home, both with the babies and without them.

## Out and About with the Kids

I originally operated under the misguided assumption that playgroups were for children. Since my newborns didn't seem to play much, I decided playgroups were not for us. This was a mistake. It turns out that playgroups are thinly disguised social networks for parents and can be great ways to find others who are not only similarly looking for interaction, but who also happen to be going through what you are. Playgroup listings can be found at libraries, online, in the newspaper, on community bulletin boards, through churches and temples, by word of mouth at the playground, or certainly through local Mothers of Twins chapters. Even if, like me, you don't think of yourself as a joiner, push yourself to go to one playgroup before you nix the idea entirely.

There is also a growing number of activities organized specifically for babies and their parents. Bear in mind that the underlying intention is simply to get you aired out a bit—to get out of the house and direct your eyes to a new scene. Don't fixate too much on the fact that your kids can't understand English yet when you weigh the value of attending a story hour at the local bookstore. The important part is that you cross the threshold of your front door and re-enter the universe outside. Here are some suggestions for things to do with the babies, if you don't have coverage for them:

- Join a gym with a nursery. Schedule a regular drop-off time in advance. Don't cancel the appointment that morning when it starts to look difficult to get everybody out of the house in one piece. Just go. Take a class or plan a decent workout.
- When you plan to take the kids out for a walk, consider mixing it up by throwing the stroller in the car and going to explore a different neighborhood or a different town. End the walk at Starbucks or a bookstore, where you can get yourself a little treat. Savor the fact that the babies are too little to clamor for treats of their own.
- Check a local newspaper for library programs, story hours, kids' musical shows, sing-alongs, and playgroups. The noise and movement of little kids and music are stimulating for the babies, and even if you don't meet your new best friend there (you might), you will have the chance to talk to other parents who are dealing with the challenges of raising little ones. Better still, you might talk about something *other than* the challenges of raising little ones.
- Some truly virtuous moms of twins that I know have found ways to take their babies with them as they do volunteer work, including spending time in nursing homes that allow helpers to bring children. I am not claiming to have exhibited this level of virtue myself, but I certainly applaud it.
- Shopping is fairly—okay, somewhat—easy at this age, once you can predict "good hours" with the babies. As long as you limit yourself to buying whatever you can cram in the bottom of the stroller, you are reasonably mobile. Sadly, malls work best, as they are climate-controlled and you only need to get in and out of the car once. But easy, girl. Remember that college tuition. And by no means should you browse for clothes for you. The idea of this trip is to help your spirits, not to deflate them entirely; you're probably nowhere near your normal size right now. Go to Crate and Barrel and spend some quality time with citrus peelers and

oven mitts, instead. Or take all those newborn clothes returns back to Baby Gap.

- If the weather is nice, hang out at the playground. No, your babies probably shouldn't attempt a full trip across the monkey bars yet, but being outdoors may knock them out and you might strike up a conversation with another mom.

## Ideas for Alone Time

You may have all sorts of ideas of what you would love to do if only you had some child care for an hour or two. But you might instead be paralyzed by the pressure to spend such precious free time well, in which case you could perhaps use a few ideas. Here are ways to spend time alone:

- Get out. Even if you just want to read a book, do it at a local coffee shop, not in bed upstairs. Get a change of scene, and experience the unbelievable ease of just hopping in the car and driving off without having to load baby equipment or perform eleven safety checks.
- About that gym...wink, wink, nudge, nudge.
- Self-spoilage: a massage, nails, facial...whatever restores you.
- Go to a movie, even if you go alone. This may feel frivolous, especially when you are paying for the movie and a sitter, but the value of the escape factor can't be exaggerated. Movies put you somewhere else entirely, and you could use a mini-vacation.
- Have lunch with someone from work. Be sure to listen closely to all her complaints about the job, so that you can be reminded of all the reasons you once looked forward to being home with babies. Purge your grass-is-greener thinking with a dose of reality. Work was stressful, too. Remember?

- Find your local chapter of the National Organization of Mothers of Twins Clubs at http://www.nomotc.org and attend monthly meetings. It's difficult to overstate the helpfulness of this group on every front, and the meetings are fun and useful.
- If it makes you happy, run errands. If it makes you irritable, don't use the time this way.
- Become a tourist in your town. Visit local art museums and historical sites that you never had time to see when you worked, other than with out-of-town visitors on the weekends. Try to hide your amazement at how easy it is to find a parking spot on a Tuesday morning.

Surely many of the suggestions above could feel frivolous relative to the intensity and importance of what is happening under your own roof right now. That's sort of the point. You need a break from that intensity, and you shouldn't worry that taking one is wasteful when in fact it is crucial to your continuing to handle the intensity of your life with baby twins. You need to feel not only the thrill of mobility but also the promise that you still exist as an individual, whole person whose identity is not formed solely around these babies. Failing to nurture yourself is one of the easiest traps to put your little paw in, and it is truly a dangerous one. You owe it to everyone—including the babies—to do whatever it takes to allow you to keep going with this project.

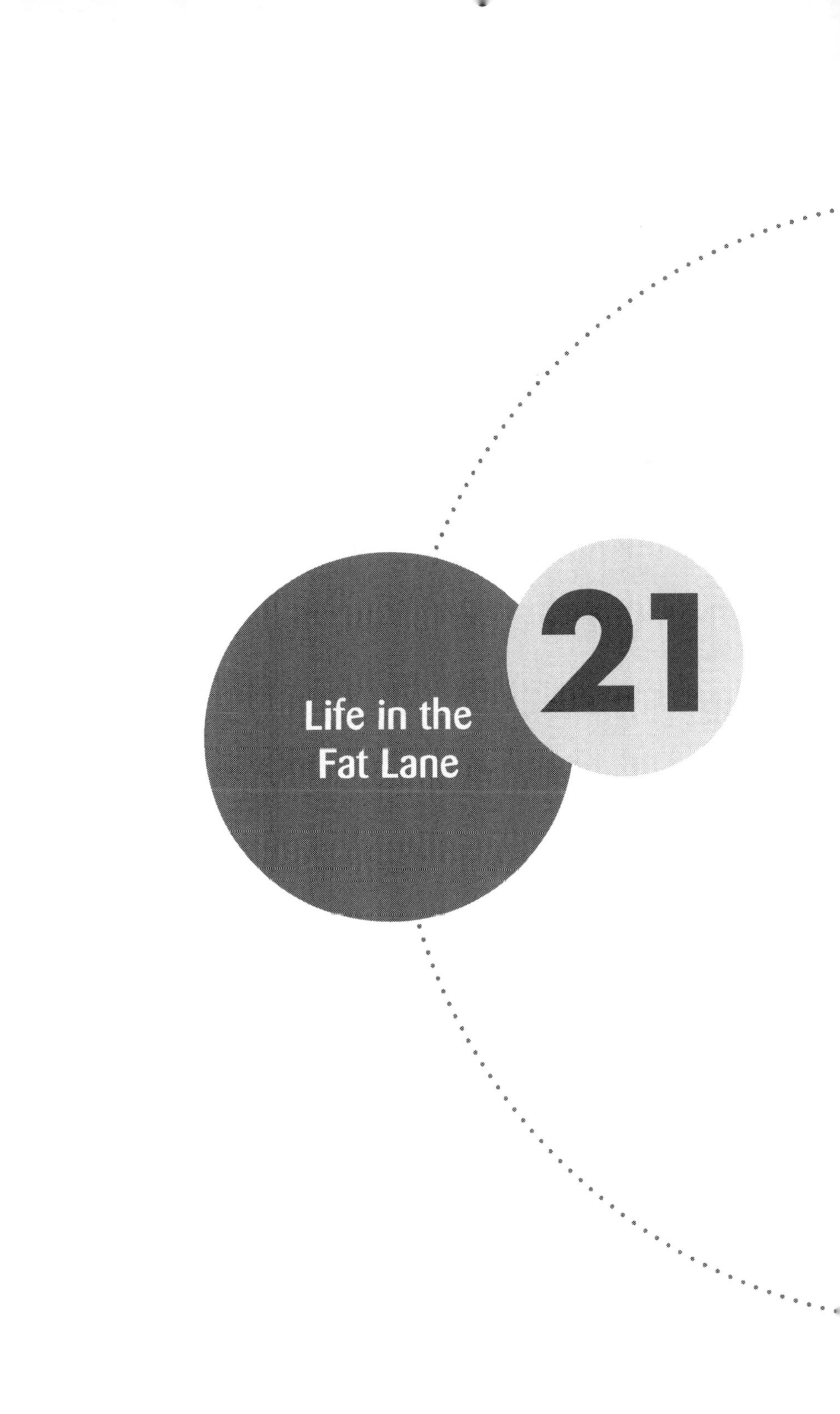
21
Life in the
Fat Lane

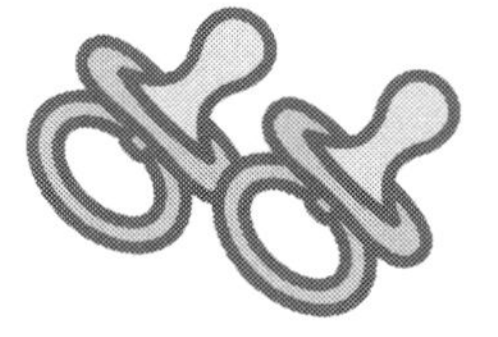

About six or eight weeks into this, there will be a moment when you manage to get a chance to take a shower and, inexplicably, as you pass the mirror, you will dare yourself to look full-on at your naked, lumpy self. Everyone else in the house will assume from the volume of your screams that a murderer had been hiding in the towel closet.

Simmer down, now. This, too, will eventually be okay. You just need to think of it in small, patient steps, and you are barely through the first one. Imagine the first three months of the twins' lives as your fourth trimester. You are still recovering from pregnancy and labor; your body is working hard to produce milk for two or is wading through a hormonal tide back to a nonpregnant, nonlactating state; your pelvis is migrating back to its original position; and generally speaking, you are beat. Where your body is concerned, your job during this period is to rest it, eat well, and begin to walk or swim or do whatever gives you energy rather than saps it. It is important that you begin to move, but you are doing so more for sanity and general health than weight loss at this point. It takes faith to look in that mirror and believe that all will be well, but it will. Not yet. But it will.

## Reality Check

I gained seventy pounds during my twin pregnancy. Let me save you the work of re-reading that: yes, *seventy*. And at the boys' first birthday, the seventy pounds were gone. But it did take the full year for that to happen. The babies were born full term at six pounds, five ounces and six pounds, eleven ounces. With another seven pounds of labor gunk left at the hospital, that was twenty pounds gone immediately. I sweated off another ten or so in the next few weeks—some from night sweats, some from terror as to how we would ever get through those first weeks. The next twenty pounds went slowly but effortlessly over six months, no doubt due in part to breastfeeding. That left twenty. And it was that remainder that had truly worried me during the pregnancy, as I knew that whether it was six pounds or forty-six, whatever I was left with after the "freebie" weight loss had leveled off was where the real work would come.

And it did take some work. Once I weaned the boys, I began to write down what I ate and shifted my habits back from the pregnancy and nursing mentality of eating enough for a tribe to my former mentality of eating enough for one—but barely. As importantly, I exercised. Not just when I had a chance. Moms of twins *never* just "have a chance" to do anything. Free time doesn't tend to pop up. Ever. Instead, exercise had to be scheduled. And then I had to stick to it. For me, running is the most efficient and effective workout, combined with lifting free weights twice a week. So starting when the twins were eight months old, I got religion about exercise. Rarely did I miss a day. It was hideously hard at first, not simply because I was achy, slow, and heavy, but because *I didn't used to be.* The difference in the experience of running from before the pregnancy to after was tough to take. Could I really have ever felt springy? Strong? Supple? Running for the first time after their birth, twenty pounds heavier and, oh yeah, a year and a half older, felt horrible. Everything hurt. I "ran" twelve-minute miles on good days, and rarely more than two or three of them at a time. I felt crunchy. And yet...

Slowly, it started feeling better. The pounds came off, perhaps a bit more reluctantly than I had hoped, but they came off. And over ten or twelve painstaking weeks, I progressed from dreading the run

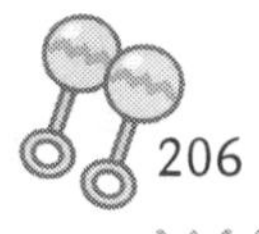


to looking forward to it to, in the end, getting bossy with my family about my right to get out every day for my workout. Once I was feeling good *during* the run and not simply *after* it, this became my coveted alone time, and I became very clever at scheduling it around the kids' bedtimes so that I could leave the most stressful scene of the day for the most relaxing one.

You need to have faith that you, too, will return to the land of the reasonably fit, even if you gained so much weight that you are unrecognizable to anyone who hasn't seen you in a year. I now know hundreds of moms of twins, and I am hard-pressed to name even one of them who has remained overweight. At some level, this is because those annoying strangers on the street who will block your double stroller to exclaim, "My, you've got your hands full!" are right. For the next few years, you will be busy, active, and much more concerned with feeding others than with feeding yourself. It may not be the healthiest solution, but the fact is that you won't have the time to overeat. As long as you don't let eating *become* a stress reliever, you are bound to lose the weight. And once you do, you will discover that you have the energy you need to take care of and play with your wonderful babies. But again, it's not time yet to panic about this. Your body is still working on this without your input.

## Breastfeeding and Weight Loss

Breastfeeding is touted as a great way to lose the baby weight, and there's certainly evidence of that. It surely burns plenty of calories. Its advantages on this front seem to come and go in stages, though. The obvious benefits kick in when your babies are between three and six months old, when the machinery of milk making is up and running at full capacity. This is the "Wow, can I eat a lot and still lose weight" stage, if you have one (not all of us do). There comes a moment in the months after that—during the second half of the babies' first year—when breastfeeding seems instead to be helping you hang on to some of the baby weight. If your body is keeping this little emergency reserve of fat (you'll find it on the back of your upper arms or squishing out of your bra—the wrong parts of your bra), it will probably drop off you like melted butter within weeks of weaning.

Everyone's body is different and reacts differently to breastfeeding. According to the National Academy of Sciences, "On average, lactating women who eat to appetite lose weight at the rate of 0.6 to 0.8 kg (1.3 to 1.6 pounds) per month in the first 4 to 6 months, but there is a wide variation in the weight loss experience of lactating women (some women gain weight during lactation)."[1] I know of plenty of women who dropped weight at rates that astonished them, and plenty who were equally astonished that they did not. In any case, it is early, and you have time. Have faith and relax about it for another month or two, at which point you'll need to start putting some modest effort in. Then, in about six months, the modest part drops away, and you've got to start working in earnest to keep the remainder from remaining.

Meanwhile, it may be hard to maintain the attitude that you hopefully achieved during pregnancy that, yes, while your newly upholstered look was sometimes disconcerting, it was all part of the mission to get two growing babies to term. Dragging your leftover weight around as those babies move through months and milestones feels a bit unfair, and it may be harder for you to see your cottage-cheesy bum as a heroic player in your kids' well-being. But it is. Well, it was, anyway. Try not to think of yourself as fat, but rather as still in the process of becoming unpregnant. Yes, it *looks* a lot like

---

1. Subcommittee on Nutrition During Lactation Committee on Nutritional Status During Pregnancy and Lactation, Food and Nutrition Board Institute of Medicine, National Academy of Sciences, *Nutrition During Lactation* (Washington, DC: National Academy Press, 1991).

fat. But the origins of your current squishiness are nobler than were the origins of your freshman fifteen. This is an honorable fat. Feel no shame.

Moreover, it is unhealthy to shed it too quickly. Losing weight rapidly is downright dangerous. You know the saying: it took nine months to put it on, it takes nine to take it off. And they're talking about a modest thirty- or thirty-five-pound gain! You probably put that much on during your second trimester alone. Nine months may not even do the trick. Don't panic. Even the weight that still clings stubbornly when you begin planning the babies' first birthday party will eventually be gone. Meanwhile, be patient with it and with yourself. As long as you are not gaining weight, you're doing just fine. Buy yourself two pairs of big-girl pants to get through the next few months and, for now, try to keep your focus on the babies' weight gains, rather than your weight losses.

# 22

# "Hey! I Was Here First!"—Sibling Rivalry

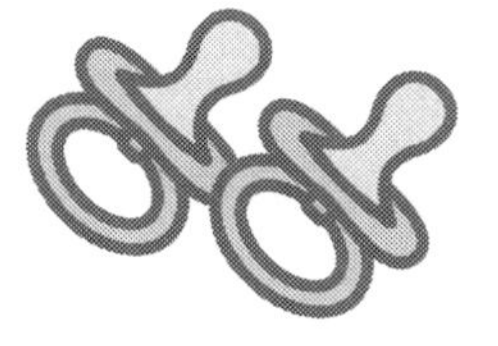

I know a fifty-year-old woman who is an identical twin. She and her sister are still cute, athletic, charming blondes (no, really…I think they're still *truly* blonde). That's an enviable laundry list for a couple of peri-menopausal dames, so imagine how irresistible they were as babies. Small wonder, then, that their six-year-old brother hated them with a pure, unwavering, unconditional sort of wrath. One can nearly forgive the little brat his indignation. After six years as prince of the palace, two little cherubs stormed the grounds on their chubby little bowed legs, overthrowing his unsuspecting reign. Lest you think this an anecdote showing how twins eventually win over even the surliest siblings, here's the sad update, half a century later: he's *still* furious with them for being born and ruining his life, and his emotional development appears to have petrified right at about the six-year mark.

There's a pretty good chance that, given the typical parenting practices of the era in which this story began, my friend's parents were less than sensitive to her brother's outrage, and might have tended to it with discipline rather than preemptive compassion. But now that we know that spanking your eldest when he feels jealous is probably *not* the best solution and may in fact lead to uneasy family holiday gatherings fifty years down the road, we need to figure out what we can do for the poor, ruined princes and princesses who find their rule usurped so unceremoniously.

Jealousy of a new baby is so predictable and natural that we have grown quite sensitive to it, and visitors are now prone to bringing

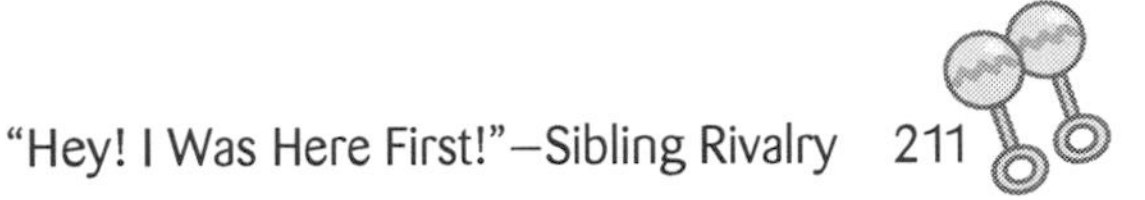

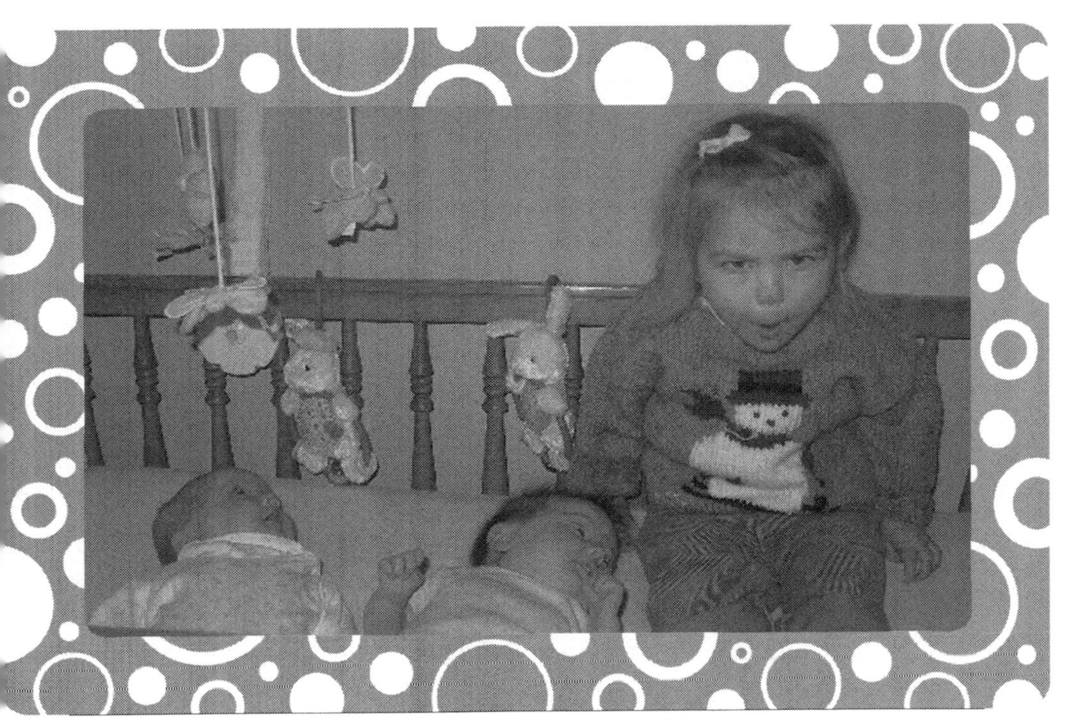

Twins can rock an older child's world, too.

Photo courtesy of the Kuchman family

big-sister or big-brother gifts when they visit newborns. Our thinking has evolved to the point that we view children as feeling creatures who respond better to understanding than chastisement. The question is how best to help an older sibling (or two or three) through jealousy and rage over the babies? The answer is laughable at this point in your life: they need more of your time.

How this issue evolves in your family will depend in large part upon the age and disposition of the older child at the time of the twins' birth. At five years old, our daughter was an unbelievable gem with the boys. She appeared to be as smitten with them as we were. It took her roughly three years to understand their ultimate threat to her place in the universe, and even then, the jealousy would flair up in little unpredictable moments of anguish that could often be easily extinguished with some one-on-one time. Jealousy is not

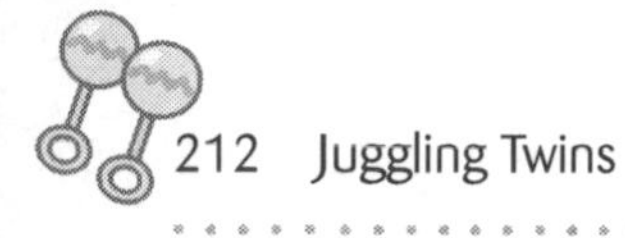


only a master of disguises that can appear as run-of-the-mill bad behavior, but for a clever child, "the jealousy card" can also become a convenient pretext for any disobedience, as in—

Mom: "Aaaaarg! Why did you draw in marker on the sofa!?"

Big Sister: (*throwing herself on the floor in feigned agony and sneaking a peek to see if it is working*) "I was jealous of the boys!"

At first, when this happened, we sat down and talked with her about her *feeeeeelings*. Soon enough, our response became, "Nice try. Get up."

In addition to feeling jealousy, older children are likely to be simultaneously proud of "their twins," and therefore may feel baffled when you are all shopping and not only have they become inexplicably invisible to strangers, but they also aren't even acknowledged as joint owners of these babies. Don't be surprised if your toddler lays his head on the babies as they are being ogled, in order to get in the picture, literally. No matter how adorable, gorgeous, or charming your eldest, there is no competing with the enchanting freak show that is twins, and there is no explaining that fact to a four-year-old, either. It is painful to witness, but can be helped by your immediate shifting of attention with a simple, "Yes, their brother is very proud of them" or, if a stranger says they are cute, offering a quick, "Yep, they look just like she did at that age." Most adults will get the hint, particularly if they are parents. Bless those who recognize the need before being reminded. I wanted to hug the grandmas who asked my daughter, "And are *you* their big sister?" as if they were asking her if she were a film star.

A co-parent can certainly make focusing on older children a priority, but the jealousy is likely to gather around mom's obvious care for and love of the twins. Sensing that she is losing you to these babies, your oldest child may want you, specifically. That's reasonable. The only way to create this time together, however, is to schedule it and get help with the babies so that you are totally freed of them and able to focus entirely on the older child. Yes, you can read a story to a preschooler while you nurse a baby, and you can even share your lap with one while you rock a baby. An older kid also needs regular time with you to herself, though, to substitute for the many hours she used to hold your full attention. Before you call the Y to schedule your oldest for three different classes to "give her something that's just hers," see if they have a class that involves both of you. The only thing she really wants that's "just hers" is you.

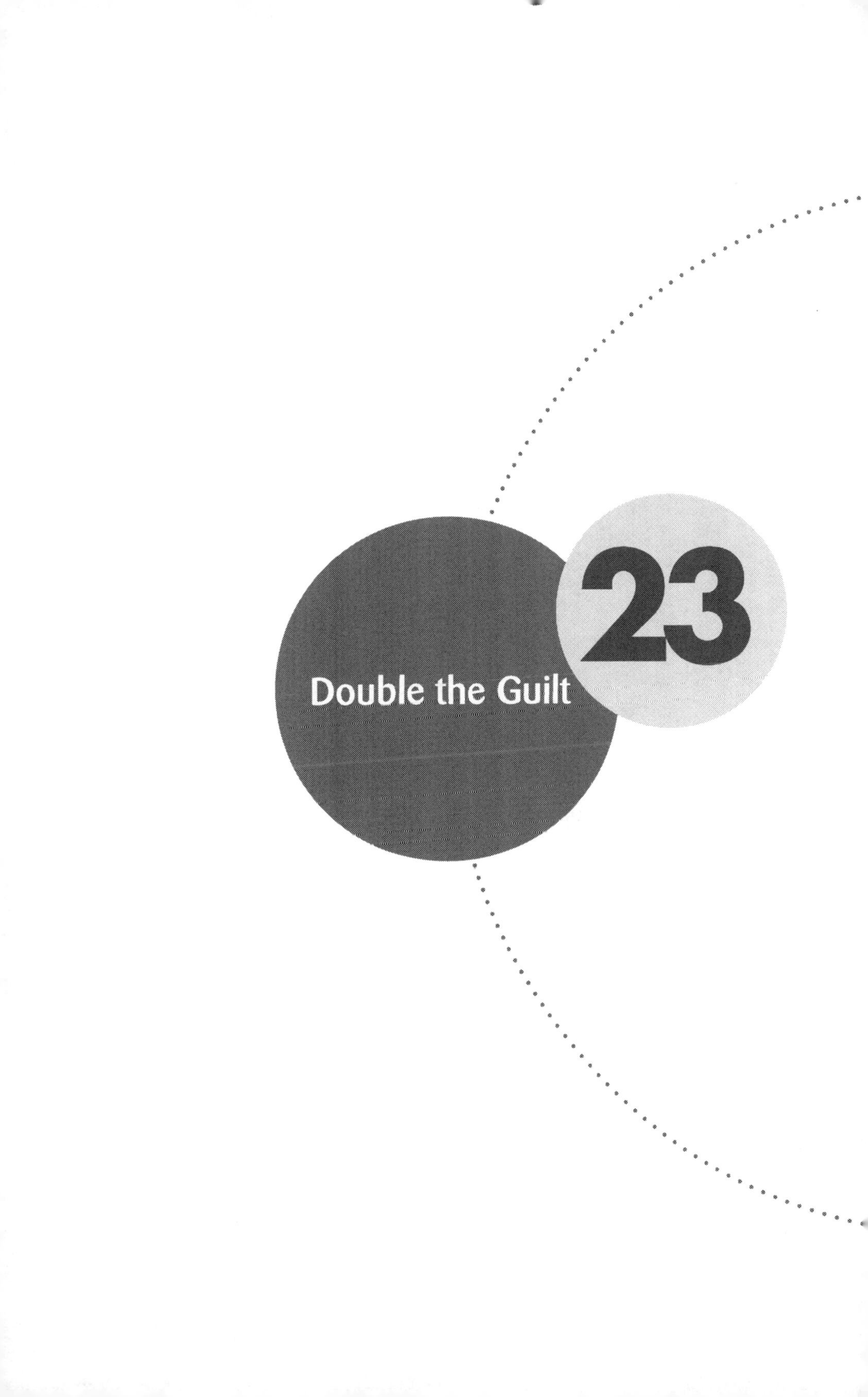

# 23 Double the Guilt

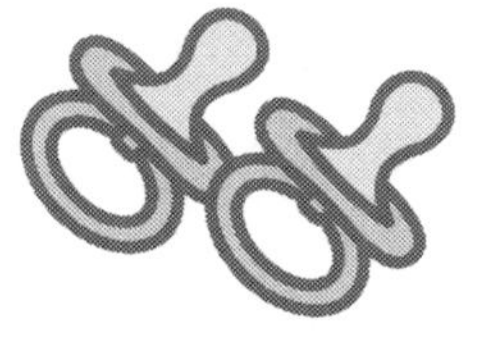

Around month three, you may begin wrestling with a nagging sense that you simply can't be as good a mother to these children as you could be to a single child. Surely, these moments are among the most difficult to cope with for a parent of twins. Consider the beauty of the design of babies. Their wails are perfectly pitched to create the effect of raising our neck hairs. Their cries can catapult our unconscious, exhausted bodies from our beds before our brains have even registered that we are now rushing urgently down a dark hall toward an ungodly screeching sound. The sound of two babies' stereophonic screeching intensifies this effect from urgency to semipanic, particularly when one is caring for the babies alone. It takes nerves of titanium to walk alone into a room in which two babies are simultaneously howling pitifully.

Months into this project, you will still face daily situations when you will gasp and wonder, "Okay, how am I going to handle this? What do I do?" There are many practical answers to that question that this book hopes to provide, but regardless of the particular strategy you adopt for each situation, there aren't always perfect solutions to answering your babies' parallel needs, and you may still at times be faced with a nagging guilt that you can't more quickly comfort and care for each child. Even if you are wealthy and able to hire so much help that your children never have to wait more than a moment for the embrace of caring arms, one child will still be in arms other than yours. You are still likely in some moments to decide that as much as you love each of them, it would have been

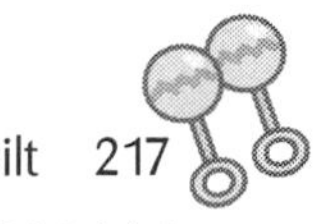

better for everyone if they had been born more than a few minutes apart. By a couple of years, perhaps.

It is healthy to acknowledge that there are elements of twinship that are imperfect and that these elements remind us that we were, by design, intended to have one offspring at a time. The most obvious effect of this reality is that often a twin will have to wait longer for comfort than a single baby would. It feels horrible not to meet a child's needs instantly; it is completely counterintuitive to allow an infant to cry, and doing so can be enormously stressful. It is not uncommon that all three—twins and caretaker—are in tears together when both babies are in distress simultaneously. In the moment, it's important to remember that you *can* comfort these babies and that eventually you will have them both settled. As one overnight caretaker once told us, "It's okay if they cry a little while. They're not in danger. They won't explode." Still, you'll have to steel yourself somewhat against your physical reaction to their crying. You are built to respond urgently but will instead have to respond calmly, methodically, and perhaps not immediately. That takes some practice.

## They're Not Blaming You

In the long run—the Big-Picture Guilt—I think it is also important to bear in mind that infant twins no more think it unjust that you split your time between them than they think it a blessing that you don't have three. Their thoughts are immediate and simple, and they have not yet developed anything remotely like a sense of fairness or a lament for your inadequacy as their parent. It is your guilt alone that tortures you over this. Later (at one year, for us), they will do their part to augment your guilt by crying or flinging themselves at your feet when you pick their sibling up for a snuggle, but even then, the gesture is not loaded with an overall sense of the injustice of their fate. It simply means, "Hey, pick *me* up!" Babies are many years away from contemplating any greener grasses of life as a singleton. Don't assign them your own baggage. They still travel light.

Your own particular flavor of self-torture may involve issues beyond the stress of not being able to meet their needs more immediately. Some of these issues may be even more acute for parents who can note contrasts with their experiences with an older singleton. Nursing one baby might have seemed a more intimate experience with your first child than nursing two together. Or you may feel, particularly in the early months, that you simply don't know your children as individuals because they have in so many senses operated as a unit. In spite of one's best efforts to obey the edict not to refer to them as "the twins" or "the girls" or even "the babies," you probably will, because it is easier and more efficient and you will be in the process of turning efficiency into an art form. And you will probably mix them up now and then, too, even if one is a thirteen-pound blonde girl and the other an eight-pound dark-haired boy, because babies are roughly the same size and shape and you are moving quickly and, sorry, but you happened to have sacrificed a *startling* number of your brain cells recently.

If yours are identical twins, you may mix them up more than you don't, and you may still be searching in vain for traits to individualize them, exaggerating any slight difference as a personality trait when in fact it could be a stage or even a mood, so desperate are you to prove to yourself that you can love each of them for him- or herself. You may even have to admit (to yourself, anyway) that you like one more than the other, much as you love them both.

*Everything* gets doubled with twins: the number of diapers, the car seats, and yes, your prescribed dosage of parental guilt.

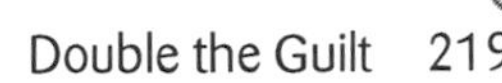

At the risk of sounding shallow and in need of therapy, my advice is to just let it go. It is simply unproductive and the facts are what they are. They are twins. That is their lot, and yes, sometimes it will not be as good a deal as it is to be a singleton, but sometimes, it will be much, much better. And their needs will be met, because you love them. They may cry a minute longer on average than their prince of an older brother had to, but who knows? They may also be refreshingly less inclined to think of themselves as royalty. And you *will* know them as individuals eventually, just not as quickly as you would with a child who is raised without another baby in the room...okay, every room. It simply takes less time to get to know one person than two. But someday you will laugh that you could ever confuse them.

Whenever I am overtaken by Multiple Guilt, feeling that surely these kids don't get enough one-on-one time, surely they won't read or speak as well as their sister did, surely they have no sense of individuality or identity and no one but their immediate family will ever be brave enough to address them by their names, I remind myself that literally every adult twin I have asked has said that he or she is happy to be a twin and wouldn't trade it for single life, given the chance. I have to believe that mine will say so, too.

# Part IV
# Months Four to Six: Okay, They Can Stay

Oh, *my,* they're cute, aren't they? Absolutely edible. Gone is the blobby, smooshy-headed splotchiness of your newborns, who even then appeared to you to be the most beautiful thing you'd ever seen, and in their places are these unbelievably adorable beings, capable of cooing and laughing at your bad jokes and sucking on their toes and each other's. And it's a good thing, isn't it? Because if that newborn period lasted much longer, the human race would have dwindled down long ago to just the six or seven crazies who truly enjoy that neonatal phase...and their children.

Let the fun begin. Bring on the faces covered in sweet potatoes and the sleeping through the night and the sitting up and giggling at each other, face to face. Bring on the stage that advertisers like to capture as having that perfect "babyness"—the big smiles and the wispy hair and the delighted squeals. Get your cameras ready, because twins can't help but be funny, and the show is about to get good. On a daily basis now, these creatures will find a hundred ways to earn their keep by charming their handlers.

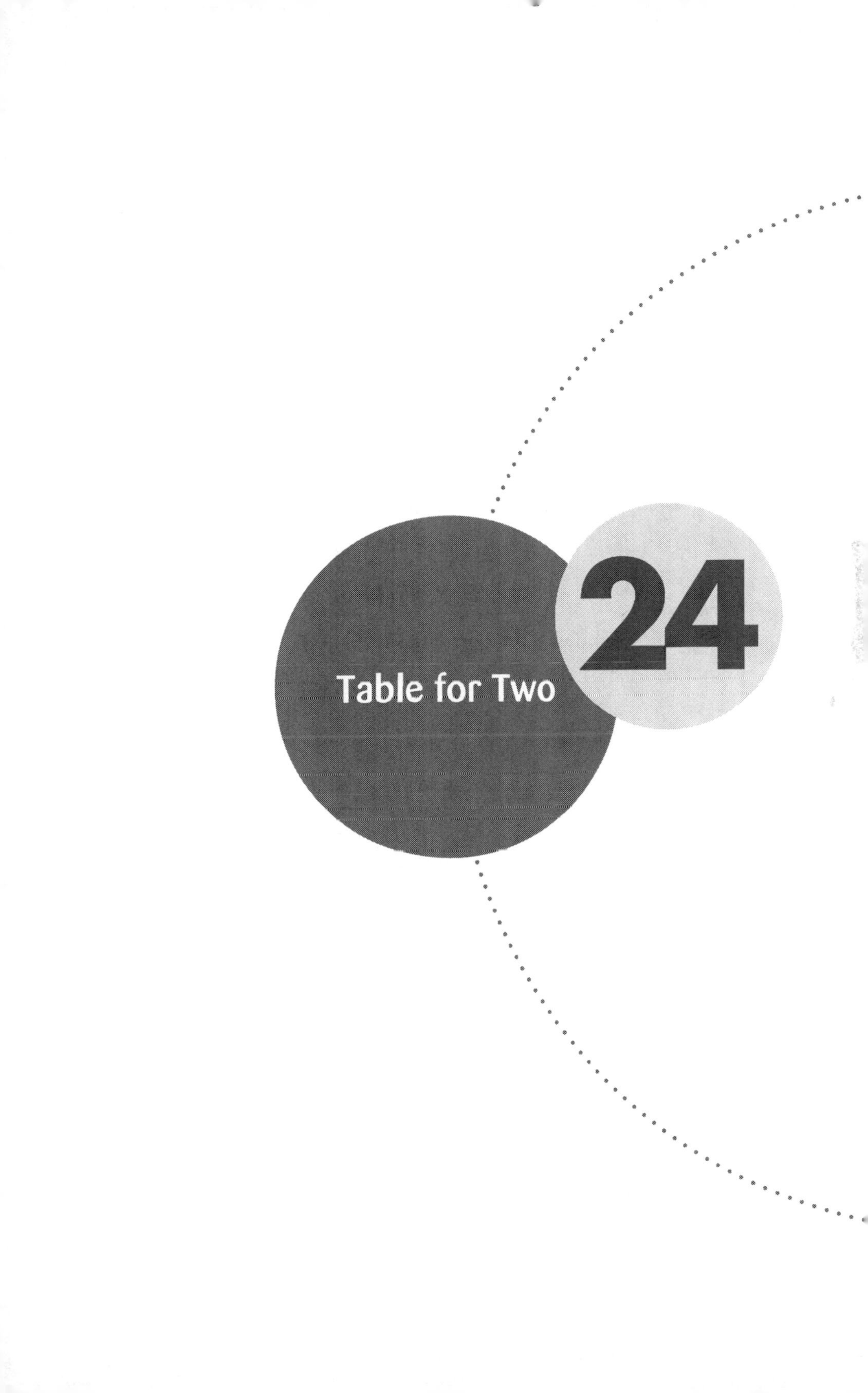
24
Table for Two

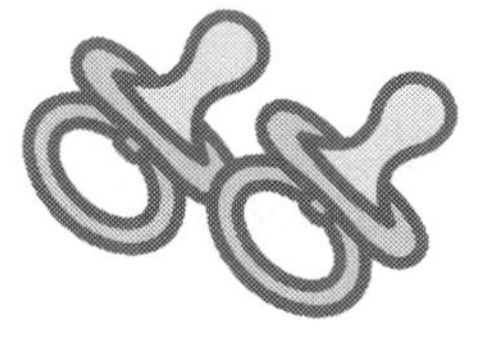

It's up to you and the babies to decide when you start solids. Chances are, you'll start them both at the same time, somewhere around the four-month mark, but there is certainly no pressure to do so; at this point, it is mostly a fun experiment. Whereas a singleton mom, just starting to feel bored by her daily baby routine, initiates a trial run with rice cereal just as soon as her baby's tongue-thrust reflex has safely faded, mothers of twins are never bored and are not likely to introduce solids simply for their entertainment value. We do get tempted, however, by the possibility that solids might produce better sleep in our kids.

Whenever you decide the magical moment has arrived, it is worth structuring it so that each child has his or her debut with solids in a solitary spotlight. This is sort of a big event, after all, worthy of some applause and a video recording when that inevitably hilarious first squished-up-in-repulsion face happens. Your twins will share at least the next several thousand meals together; during their first few weeks of eating, they should have the experience and your attention to themselves. Since they can't sit up yet, each will enjoy being held by you as you feed him. You will by now have read all the baby operating manuals that teach you to introduce rice cereal first, followed perhaps by barley or oatmeal, then the fruits, right on through the list until they are happily sawing away at beef jerky. Introducing solids is a fun rite of passage that is fairly straightforward, especially in that first month, when nutrition takes a back seat to education as the object of eating.

## Setting Up the Kitchen

Once your twins can sit up without slumping over like cowboys that just got shot in their seats at the saloon, you've all entered a new world. The high chair or its equivalent means that the babies now have the ability to eat more like real people. They have a new place for playing and two trays on which you can place all sorts of interesting distractions. It is a real graduation for them, as it means that a play space has finally moved up off the floor and into the world of big people. The trouble is that you need to have a very large kitchen indeed in order to be able to fit and maneuver around two space-hogging high chairs.

If your kitchen is less than a quarter acre in area, you may want to consider a few other options. The first is those very cool, collapsible high chairs that stack like giant card-table folding chairs. Another is the old-fashioned hook-on seats that pop the kids right onto the side of a sturdy table or a counter with a protruding edge. We loved our inherited Graco Tot-Loc chairs; they were probably ten years old, but they worked great and took up no floor space. With them appended to an island in the center of the kitchen, we could face the kids and reach right over the counter to feed them. There are all sorts of new options, too, including fabric braces that slip over the back of a normal chair and hold the baby securely in place as she eats at the table. Weigh your options before you invest the time or space in high chairs. You may not need them at all.

## Introducing Solids: The Three Phases

1. The Learning Stage, when each of them needs your help individually and you are gradually introducing a variety of new foods and waiting a couple of days between each one in order to watch for allergies. (Write reactions down! You'll eventually forget who ate what and what reaction occurred.)

2. The Creamed or Smashed Everything Stage, when you are painstakingly spoon-feeding both of them, probably simultaneously, and then mopping the place up afterward.
3. The Hallelujah Stage, when after spoon-feeding them a bit of strained stuff, you can put some finger food down in front of them and saunter across the room to start the dishes.

The four-to-six-month period is still firmly planted in the first stage. A baby will usually be able to sit up to eat at about six or seven months, but the spoon-feeding will go on for a number of months after that.

My goal was to move as swiftly as possible from stage one straight through to stage three, and my strategy was essentially to *make finger food out of the mushy foods* and deal with the consequences later. The dogs became instrumental players in this plan and gained approximately seventeen pounds each in three months, all on splatterings of oatmeal and bits of banana from the floor. While moms with only one kid might have focused on bonding with their babies at this time of day, my focus was beginning to shift toward regaining control of the household, starting with scaling the mountain of daily dishes. The twins' meals became somewhat productive times for me. Food could keep them entertained for a good, long stretch.

In the process of becoming ever more efficient, we also learned that we needed lots of bibs so that we always had clean ones. Eventually, we also learned that each bib needed a safety pin at the back, because they tried to pull the Velcro ones off—themselves *and* each other. We had a giant basket of bibs and stacks of single-ply cotton diapers that served as baby face wipes and then, folded over, as counter wipes.

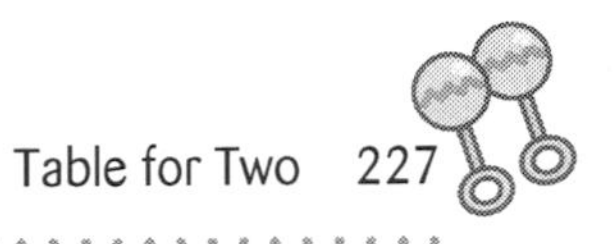

## Great Foods to Start With

You'll notice an absence of processed foods in the following list of great mushy-fingery foods for babies. Here's my reasoning: your babies' interest in food will never be unspoiled again, so why develop in them a predilection for salt or sugar when they still think that plain, cold tofu is a marvel?

### Finger-Food Ideas (All Smooshed and/or Served in Small Bits)

Plain, cold tofu

Egg yolks, cooked and crumbled (no whites yet)

Shredded cheese

Bits of veggie burger

Fish (not tuna or other "steaky" fishes)

Whole-wheat macaroni

Cut-up toast bits with hummus

Orzo

Chickpeas (mash 'em up well)

Avocado

Peas (run frozen ones under hot water)

Sweet potato

Mashed potato

Steamed carrots

Lima beans or edamame, peeled

Green beans, cooked and cut small

Acorn squash, baked

Mashed cauliflower

Frozen mango or berries (hold off on strawberries)

Banana

Cooked apples

Very ripe pear

The ubiquitous Cheerios

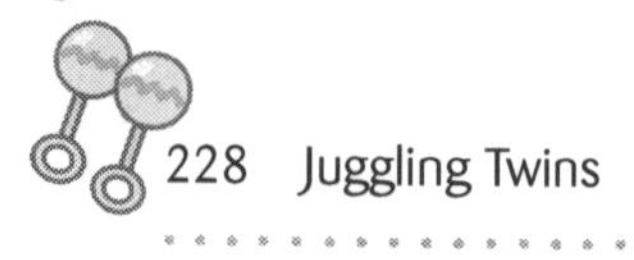


Don't stress yourself yet about attaining perfect nutritional balance at every meal. Your babies still get all they need in liquid form, and the entire idea at this point is to teach them the simple pleasure of eating wholesome foods in the company of people we love. Surely, that clump of sweet potato you find in your hair an hour after lunch won't diminish the beauty of that stirring life lesson even a smidgen.

# 25

# Sleep Training Two...Or Not

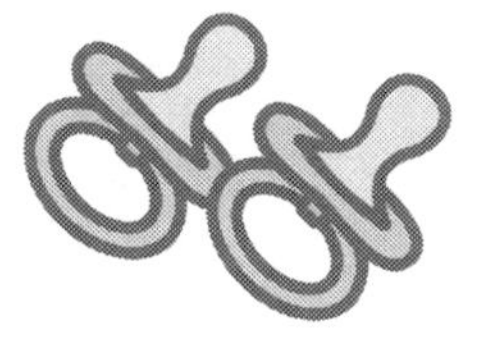

If you are of the opinion that allowing babies to cry is just too awful to contemplate, I respect you. I also pity you, however, because the next couple of years—or more—will be exceedingly tough for you and yours. Yes, it is painful to listen to your babies' cries and stand still. It flies in the face of every instinct you have as a mother, actually, and you will likely be filled with self-doubt in the moment even if you were filled with resolve when you began. But dealing with erratic sleep—their sleep and yours—for the next several *years* is in my opinion far worse and far more damaging than a couple weeks of hell. Interestingly, the debates about sleep training on twin message boards are not like those on general parenting boards. The question seems not to be "Should we do it?" but "*When* should we do it?" or "Can we start yet? Please?" Teaching twins to sleep well is a very basic survival strategy for parents of twins.

If you are in agreement with this basic premise, then you should read and adopt a full approach, rather than just boiling the message down to letting the kids scream at night.[1] It's a bit more involved and should be done with planning and care. As with everything, there are several complicating factors with twins. The most obvious is that once they are through the newborn period, twins sleeping in the same room can wake each other with crying. If you don't have a spare bedroom in which you can temporarily set up another crib or Pack-n-Play, then set one up in your own bedroom. The normal stresses of sleep training

1. Since Richard Ferber and Marc Weissbluth initiated the debate, plenty of authors, researchers, and "baby whisperers" have thrown their hats in the ring on this question. There's a multiplicity of approaches to sleep training, and it's worth investigating a few of them before you choose a plan.

are compounded inordinately when, just as a baby has finally gotten herself to sleep, she is awakened by her twin's crying. The farther you can get the babies apart, the better, so that they can't even hear each other down the hall. This arrangement will be short-lived, and you'll be able to return them to a shared room once they have gotten the idea. It might also be a good idea to have them take turns in the adjunct room, so that each baby experiences putting himself to sleep in his own crib. Later on, your twins will not be fazed in the least by the nighttime crying of the other, but during this period, it can be a real problem.

## Reality Check

With our first child, the question of whether and how to sleep train—to allow some amount of crying in the name of teaching her to get herself to sleep—was all-consuming. There seemed at the time to be a great debate afoot among parents as to the best approach: was it cruel to allow babies to cry in order to get them to sleep better? Plenty of online moms seemed to think so, and argued that it was simply unnatural not to go to a crying child, no matter the time of night and no matter how many times per night. Others said no, what was cruel was setting a child up for a lifetime of sleep issues and perhaps allowing her to be in a constant state of overtiredness due to her inability to consolidate her sleep.

We read all the books and, when our daughter was five months old, decided to "Ferberize" her—the common misnomer for "crying it out," based on the name of one of the first authors to address this issue in a full-length book.[2] The method we chose was actually Marc

*continued...*

2. Richard Ferber, *Solve Your Child's Sleep Problems,* 1st Fireside Edition (Simon & Schuster, Inc., 1986). Ferber's detailed plan has been sadly oversimplified as CIO, or "cry it out," and parents tend now to refer any plan to sleep train as "Ferberizing" their child.

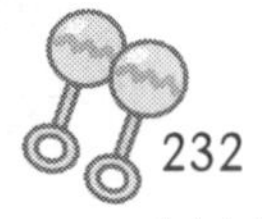


Weissbluth's, from his book *Healthy Sleep Habits, Happy Child.*[3] It worked like a charm. Our eldest became an amazing sleeper, and we became ardent advocates of earlier bedtimes, regimented naps, and yes, occasional crying it out in the name of teaching her to self-soothe and consolidate her sleep hours. Five years later, as avowed converts, we knew from the start that we would sleep train our twins.

When sleep training, remember some of the basics of getting good sleep from your babies. Darken the windows in both rooms with blackout material or double drapes. Use white noise; employ bedtime routines religiously. Swaddle your babies if they'll still allow it. With most programs, you will probably start with nighttime put downs and graduate to naps. (The process of getting twins to nap well occupies its own special level in Sleep Hell. Skip ahead to "Napping Nightmares..." if you can't stand the suspense.)

If baby sleep issues consume parents of single babies, then they threaten to swallow parents of twins whole. It is extremely hard work getting twins to sleep regularly and dependably. The vast consensus among experienced mothers of twins is that the awful work of sleep training is both more horrible and more important with twins. But the news isn't all bad. If, for example, you have identical twins, you may find that their sleep patterns are remarkably similar. Our twins were inclined to sleep for the exact same duration even when they slept on opposite sides of the house. Their tendency to wake within one minute of each other was downright uncanny and convinced me that they were emitting "awake" vibes across the house. This made it easier to get them on a schedule; they were naturally in sync. And while some parents find hideous the idea of staying home every morning and afternoon in order to protect their baby's naptime, hey, you're already home! You can barely get out of the house as it is.

---

3. Marc Weissbluth, *Healthy Sleep Habits, Happy Child* (Random House, 2003).

Finally, when all of this madness is finished and you have two great little sleepers, having two in the same room will actually buy you a few *more* minutes of sleep in the morning. There's nothing better than hearing your babies happily yammering away to each other when they wake up in the morning. Ours could (and still do) entertain each other as we seized a few more minutes of drowsy, drifty sleep. The first time that happened may have been our moment of realizing that we were going to let them stay.

# 26

# One Sick, Two Sick (Three Sick, Four)

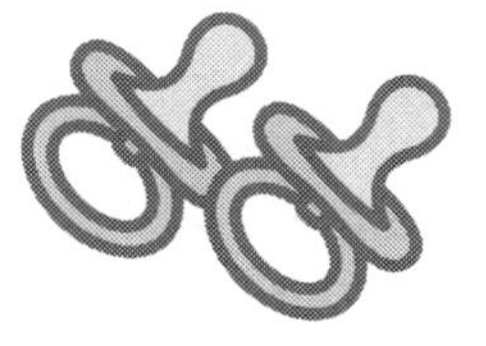

After you have managed to make it through the newborn months, nothing will bring you straight back to those days faster than a virus. When your kids are sick, all of you revisit the infant period not only in terms of the babies' collective neediness, but also in terms of what the nights look like and how you are pretty sure you won't be able to muddle through them. The only differences are an added layer of worry and the fact that, unlike with the newborn stage, sickness comes unannounced and always at the least convenient time. You will get to the point that, when you hear a child sniffle three rooms away, you will mechanically scan your next four days' worth of appointments, knowing that all of them are now in peril.

Even before your babies can play together, they will generously share with each other their every bug. Colds never stop at the first baby, perhaps because you yourself are such a marvelous transport system between them, kissing and cuddling them each as you do. Other children in your family may be spared but probably won't be and are usually the prime suspects for bringing the viruses home in the first place. In all, when a wave of sickness appears on the horizon, you need to go back into drop-everything mode, and this can be much more difficult now that you are all in the rhythm of a routine than it was when the babies were just born and you had already dropped everything. And of course, there's a pretty good chance that you feel crappy too and could stand a little mothering yourself.

Treat the first signs of illness as you would the first report of a major snowstorm on the way. Because it will be very hard for you to get out of the house once this storm has arrived, check at the start to see that you have enough food, acetaminophen and ibuprofen, and Gatorade to allow you all to hunker down for a few days if necessary. When colds and coughs hit, it may also be best to separate twins who share a room, not because it will keep them from spreading it—it won't—but because nighttime coughing can keep a non-cougher up.

A dear friend of mine whose "babies" now have their own babies has always said that she liked her kids best when they were sick. She raised three fiery, independent daughters and enjoyed those moments when, for a short while, they were needy, red-cheeked little urchins curled in her arms, wanting only their mama. For her, however, the scene was not complicated by the wails of another child across the room, wanting only *his* mama.

Having sick twins creates one of those familiar scenarios in which you will feel that there just isn't enough of you to mother properly. It is heart wrenching not to be able to go immediately to a sick child, even if your reasons are sound. Try telling a crying kid with a temp of 102.5 degrees and a sore throat that he'll have to wait to be held because you are presently rushing a vomiting sibling down the hall to the bathroom.

The aftermath of illness is also tougher with two. Just when you seem to have a tentative hold on this sleep-training business, a stomach bug can come through and blow the whole thing to shreds, making you start all over again. Clearly, sick children may or may not stick with the sleep plan and will probably need to be coddled in the middle of the night. It takes merely two minutes of midnight rocking for a baby to decide she can no longer sleep through the night without being rocked on the hour, and this reversal of sleep training always outlasts the virus. Back to square one.

# 27

# Twinproofing the House

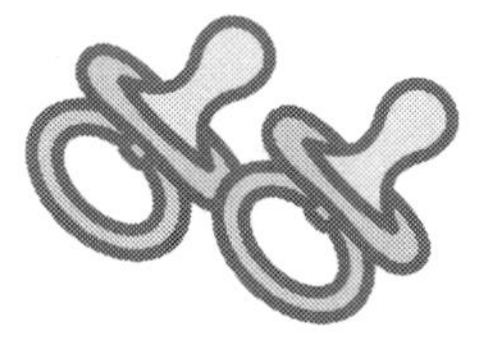

If these are your first babies, the baby manuals you have read may have convinced you to have your home entirely babyproofed by the time you start to show. If these are not your first, you may have waited longer, having remembered that those plastic covers on your electrical sockets served only to irritate you and break your fingernails until your baby was about six or seven months old, at which point they became nearly useful, as the kid was giving occasional thought to scooting in the general vicinity of a socket.

> We are an anxious generation, so convinced that a disaster will happen on our watch that some savvy women are now marketing themselves as "babyproofing consultants." For a handsome fee, they will come into your home to point out all the unanticipated ways in which your house could do in your baby.

This is not something you need to concern yourself with until the babies are quite mobile, because at the beginning of their motoring, you're not going to be letting them out of your sight for an instant, anyway. Once they are on the move, however, you do need to get on it in a proactive manner, rather than with a "let's see what interests them and then secure it" approach. Whereas parents of singletons tend to babyproof the entire home and let the baby have a fairly long leash in her wanderings, having two new crawlers on the loose is an unsettling vision, no matter what the level of security. What if you *lose* one?

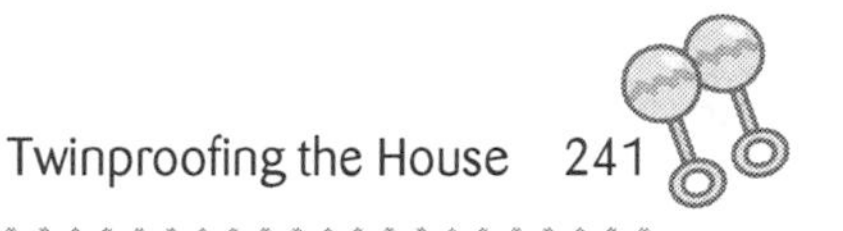

## The Corral

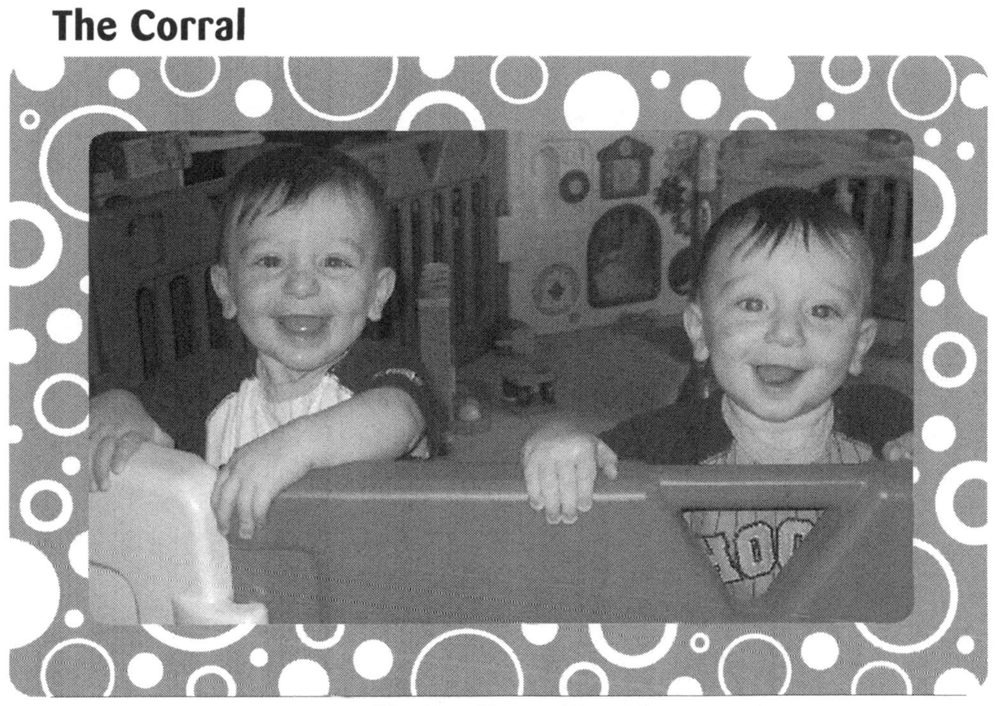

"The Corral"—round 'em up!

Photo courtesy of the Goldberg family

By the time your kids can sit up, you need to have begun getting them used to the notion of *containment*. Borrow every playpen, play yard, and superyard you can get your hands on, so that you can start small and expand their area as their size and skills increase. At four to six months, plop them together in a crib or a regular-sized playpen several times a day with a toy or two for ten-to-fifteen-minute periods. At this point, you'll still need to supervise them fairly carefully. By the time they are six to eight months old, sitting up reliably and beginning to crawl, they will be used to this idea of hanging out with each other in a cordoned-off area. What's more, you'll be able to allow them to play safely in their "corral" for much longer than could the parent of a singleton—and with less guilt, as they will happily hang out together, swap toys, and little by little begin to play with each other.

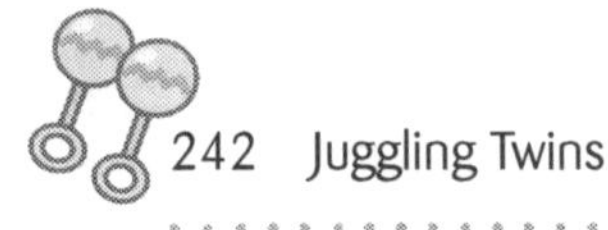



A singleton baby unceremoniously dumped to languish for hours in a playpen while his mother watches *Oprah* has been a lamentable image in the view of many parenting experts, and it's a justifiable point. But twins in a contained play area create a different scenario altogether, diminishing the increased risks associated with having two babies on the loose and stimulating each other with increasingly complex interactions.

## Reality Check

By the time our guys were nine months, they had initiated games of "chase," giggling as they pursued each other around an eight-by-eight-foot play area in a hilarious *über-crawl* that got them going so fast at times that their legs would come out from under them. By ten months, they worked on stacking cups together and passed toys back and forth, and by one year, they rolled a ball back and forth between themselves. The incidents of gouged eyes, full-out tackles, and hurt feelings were remarkably few (but don't forget to keep nails cut short), and our "pigpen" became indispensable to us not simply as a safe baby depository but as a fun place for them to explore and learn. Ours was smack in the center of things, close to the front door, so that they were always in the thick of activity, rather than sequestered to a quiet corner.

If you have or can create enough space, try to get hold of enough panels or extenders so that you can make their primary play area at least six feet by six feet. Remove a piece or two of furniture from a central room for these months if necessary to create a big enough parcel for them. That way, their sense of confinement will be lessened, and the area will also be inviting for bigger folks and siblings to hop in and play with the babies. From six months on, babies will love to have a bigger family member simply lie in their space to serve as a mountain to crawl up and over. Pig-piles in the pigpen became our favorite leisure activity during these months, and it was not uncommon to find the entire family in the pen, lolling about and playing.

If your home has two stories, try to find space for a second, smaller play area upstairs, so that the babies can have some variety and you can have a safe spot for them when you need to be upstairs. This second pen is also useful when you are taking babies up to their room, allowing you to safely carry one upstairs and leave her in the upstairs pen while you fetch her twin from the downstairs pen. Ideally, you will have a large space for them downstairs, an auxiliary space upstairs, and a fully—I mean *fully*—babyproofed nursery where you feel safe putting one on the floor while you change the other's diaper or clothes, or sing one to sleep while the other plays for one last minute on the floor. Some twin parents install "Dutch doors" on the nursery (that is, *they saw the door in half*), but it will work just as well to put a gate up across their door frame, even if it needs to be removed regularly. My household feels enough like a barnyard already; swinging doors won't help things. Ideally, the nursery should approximate a padded cell as nearly as possible.

The keys to making these play spaces good experiences for your kids are to resist the temptation to overuse them totally—as in, all day—and to rotate in new toys and activities regularly. Having fewer toys helps them focus and also keeps the area uncluttered enough so that they can move about freely and work on their crawling, cruising, and eventually walking. Having too many toys in their space will frustrate them as much as having too few.

Try to anticipate fussiness rather than react to it after the fact. Keep ten or twelve toys—not all thirty—in the area, and remove a couple and replace them with something new every ten or fifteen minutes.

Depending on their age, you will be able to get quite a lot done when they are happily and safely frolicking in their pen. When they are six months old, you can bring a basket of laundry out to fold in the same room. At one year, they may even be able to be monitored through the opening to the next room—perhaps from the kitchen as you prepare their next meal. At every age that you use a pen with them, though, get in the habit of surveying the floor area before you pop them in. This is particularly important if you have older children who may have dropped a tiny Polly Pocket shoe or Lego piece in, but even if there aren't older kids, you'll want to check for errant dust balls, leaves that came in on someone's shoes, or buttons that popped off a shirt. Scan it every time you go to use it.

If you find the idea of confining your kids in this manner repugnant, well, God bless and good luck. You're in for it. Buy disposable clothing for your family and count on lots of take-out meals for the next six months. Supervising two babies who have constant free rein, regardless of the level of babyproofing in your home, is a very intense proposition and one that requires that you not urinate when the babies are awake. So ask yourself: am I really ready for adult diapers? As a seventy-five-year-old mother of seven and grandmother of twenty-five told me upon meeting my twins when they were six months old, "Cage them *now*. You'll never get them in there once they've tasted freedom."

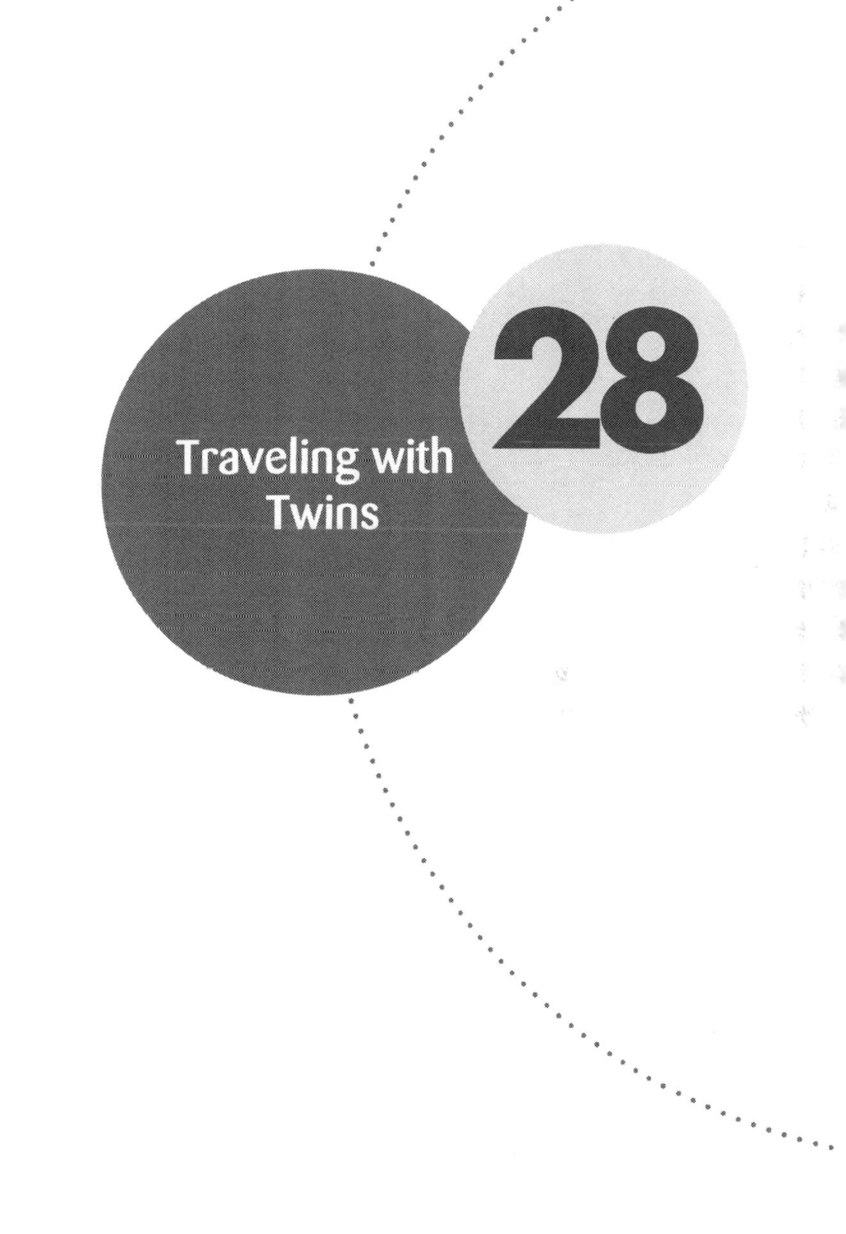

# 28

# Traveling with Twins

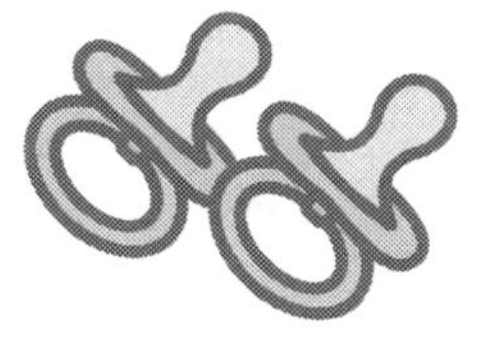

If you have flipped forward to this topic from very early chapters because you have an impending trip, there's good news. In some ways, traveling with newborns is much easier than traveling with older babies or toddlers. The period between six months and two years is probably the toughest for traveling with twins, but every age is doable, and you should not feel grounded until further notice. Some strategizing is called for, however, depending upon your situation.

## Flying

On most airlines, booking seats for babies is optional up to the age of two. The age of your children and the number of adults traveling will both play roles in this decision. Because the bargain of flying babies for free is so tempting and because, with two, the difference between buying and not buying can now mean many hundreds of dollars, a lot of parents of twins don't book seats and instead hold out hope that there will be empty seats on the plane, which gate clerks are usually more than willing to make available to families at takeoff. But when was the last time you were on a flight that wasn't full? If you want to try this approach, you can increase your chances of free seats by booking at unpopular times—very early in the morning or very late at night, preferably midweek. Doing so affords you another advantage, too, which is the slightly reduced stress level in a plane that's not packed to its wings with grumpy passengers staring down your twins with their "not next to me, please" eyes as you board.

If you are nervous about the possibility of having no empty seats available, you can always buy one ticket and take one car seat on in order to allow one baby to hang out in it while you hold the other. Some airlines offer half-price fares for babies. This is a good option, too, if you are traveling alone with the twins, since you obviously can't hold two in your lap for the flight.

Another consideration when purchasing tickets is that if you have two adults traveling with twins and another child, you will have to split up into different rows, even if you plan to hold the babies. There aren't enough oxygen masks in one row for five people. If you have to schedule connecting flights and have a choice about your second leg, be sure to leave plenty of time between flights. It is better to hang out in the airport and regroup than try to sprint through three terminals with your entire caravan. Even if you are a speedy group, you may have to wait a while for your gate-checked equipment to be returned to you.

## What to Bring

In planning what gear to bring, think about what you will be checking and what you will be taking all the way to the gate. We tended to take one giant bag on rollers with all our collective clothes, and we would do a curbside check of that and the Pack-n-Plays. The stroller and car seats we took all the way to the gate—the stroller for our own convenience and the car seats in case there were empty seats for babies on the plane. (This makes those car-seat travel covers a waste of money. Car seats are sturdy and their padding is washable, anyway.) Some mothers of twins have suggested that Baby Joggers, though bigger, are better choices than strollers because they are taken around the security scanners to be checked manually, which relieves you of the hassle of unloading, folding, and placing a stroller on the conveyer. Just be sure you can fold it at the gate.

Another possibility, particularly if you're not the only adult, is to bring two cheap umbrella strollers and a connector. If your kids are

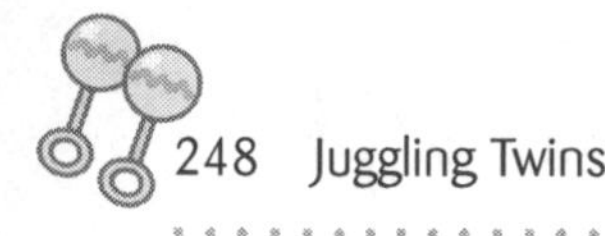


still in infant car seats, check the instructions before you travel to ensure that they are designed to (and that you know how to) buckle them in without the bases; the seats for babies over 22 pounds are secured in the plane the same way they are in your car. There is also a product on the market called Baby B'air that harnesses kids into your lap. It runs about $30 and is for use during flight, not during takeoff and landing. Reviews haven't been great on these, though, relative to the expense. We used our Baby Bjorns in this way and they worked fine.

Depending on where you're going, you will probably need a Pack-n-Play or two for the twins to sleep in during the trip. If you have joined the Mothers of Twins club, you know that you can post online requests on message boards of the group in your destination area and are likely to find someone very willing to lend you theirs, or even a spare crib or two. If you are going to Grandma's house and plan to do so regularly, you might want to check craigslist in her area or put her on the project of hunting down yard sales in order to get two used portable cribs for her house so that you can simply eliminate the Pack-n-Plays from your packing list. It's probably worth it if you'll visit more than once and she's willing to store them for you. There are also websites that allow you to order baby supplies for your destination point while traveling so that you don't need to carry everything with you (see Resources section). If that seems extravagant, you should at least feel comfortable asking whomever you are visiting to do a shopping run for you so that you have baby food, diapers, formula, and whatever else you need waiting for you when you arrive.

## Getting through Security

TSA now allows women to bring "reasonable amounts" of breast milk or formula through security as carry-on items (and no, you won't have to swig some of it to prove it's not explosive). Nonetheless, it may be easier to bring premeasured formula mix packs if your babies use formula. You can always buy bottled water on the other side of security or get it from the flight attendant. Baby bottles with liners provide easier clean-up when you travel. If you don't have any and don't want to buy new bottles, remember to bring some dish soap (under three ounces) in a small bottle, and perhaps a bottle brush. Don't forget to put all liquids in a plastic bag, including baby food (also allowable). Bring healthy snacks for everyone. We always wrap two small new toys per kid for opening and playing with *en route*. Try to limit carry-on items to what you and the babies absolutely must have during the trip, plus a change of shirts for everybody and two pairs of pants for the babies, just in case. Don't fool yourself by carrying on your book or *People* magazine. There will be other trips for that. You'll be moving two children, a stroller, and two car seats. Add to that as little as you can in order to get by. If you put a small pack of wipes and a handful of dipes in a big plastic bag, you can take just this and a baby to the bathroom to change, rather than the whole diaper bag.

When travel day arrives, wear clogs or other slip-ons so that you don't have to re-tie your shoes after you're through security. When dressing the twins, remember that you may need to play the twin card for all it's worth. Dress them adorably, and if you can stand it, consider matching outfits. For once, you *want* to draw attention to the twins, so that you can get all the help and sympathy possible. It's finally time to rip the tags off those matching sailor suits! When you plan your transportation to the airport, remember that many of the shuttles that take you from remote parking lots don't have seat belts for the car seats. It might be worth asking a friend to drop you all off. Once there, security is the biggest hassle. In order to pass through, you will have to disassemble your carefully packed bag, take the children out of the stroller, and somehow walk through the scanner with only one of them at a time. This is the break-a-sweat moment if you are the only adult here. In either case, though, relax, take your

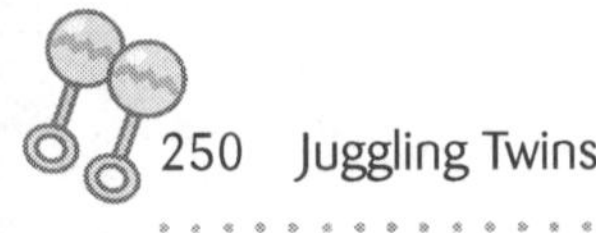



time, and focus, so that nothing (and nobody) gets left behind. If the corporate types behind you are huffing their coffee breath down your neck because their flight is boarding, it's their own fault for leaving the house late. You don't need to feel pressured.

Once you are through the rigmarole, be sure to check your bags twice to make sure nothing is missing. When you get to the gate, see if you will have a preboarding option. Be sure the clerk can see the sailor suits as you ask, and if you can make your voice quiver a bit, all the better. If there is no preboard option, it might then be best to get on the plane last. If there are two adults, one can get on with all the equipment and get it set up while the other waits five or ten minutes and then brings the babies on. Change both babies right before boarding; it's tough to change diapers on a plane. Once on, grab a bunch of pillows in case your back hurts from holding a baby in your lap. Have pacifiers ready for takeoff, to help with ear discomfort. Don't stress out when your babies cry. So they're crying. So *what?* The majority of flyers are parents and have been through it and are mostly just relieved that the screamer isn't theirs. You have enough stress and don't need to worry about your fellow passengers today.

## Car Trips

Perhaps this is just nostalgia talking, but it seems like road trips used to be less stressful. That was back before people started using their cars as phone booths, drifting in and out of your lane as they scroll through their cell phone contact list. Road trips are still easier with kids than flights, though, if for no other reason than you have some control over the situation and can bail and head to a hotel at any point if it becomes too unbearable. We have had some great car trips with our kids, including several trips from the East Coast to Michigan and back with infants and a kindergartener. Traveling by car spares you the agony of cancelled flights and exposure to the viruses that thrive on airplanes, and it requires no security check or especially careful packing.

And there's just nothing like a long trip to get you singing the praises of diapers. A kid can go hours in those things with no need to stop. (I know what you're thinking, but don't try it...Depends will definitely make you look fat.) Bring lots of great snacks, new toys, a stack of books with flaps, and some kid music. You might want to borrow DVD players for anyone over a year old. Be willing to stop as often as necessary to keep you all happy. Again, this is not a race. Plan departure times for naptime or bedtime. Theirs, not yours. Consider volunteering to drive first. Once you see how busy the kids keep your adult passenger with dropped books and the need for snacks, you will realize that driving is infinitely easier. I have been known to say, "No, I'm fine, I'll keep driving" all day, at every stop, eventually putting in twelve hours at the wheel rather than ride shotgun.

# Part V
# Months Seven to Twelve: Breathing Again

A woman recently asked me when the "tipping point" was with our twins—when the advantages of having twins kicked in. In trying to answer, I realized that there are two key milestones in the emergence of benefits in having twins. The first is when they can entertain each other in a manner that a single baby cannot do for herself, giving you occasional breaks from keeping baby happily occupied that singleton moms don't get. The second milestone, which is a huge one, is the moment when the advantages of having twins actually begin to outweigh and offset the trials of having them. The first milestone happens in the six-to-nine-month range. The second one happens a couple of years later and involves not only their having a permanent playdate, but also the conveniences of shared vaccination and annual physical schedules, the same or similar team obligations and swim lessons, the possible sharing of clothes, the occasional price break when signing both up for programs, and in general, shared needs at approximately the same time, unlike most siblings, whose needs are developmentally staggered.

For now, you can begin to savor the conveniences of having two when you see that they can play happily together for a much longer time than can one baby plopped in a playpen with an assortment of toys. You just don't get the sort of giggles from one baby with a rattle that you do from two babies rolling all over each other like puppies, and that fun is here to stay for at least a few years. Slowly, the other advantages will now begin to accumulate like a slow drip of congratulatory rewards for your having run the gauntlet of raising twin babies. You are moving through the hardest part and should find among your prizes a bit more sleep, a light at the end of the tunnel, and two adorable babies whose daily charms continue to earn them room and board.

# 29

# Dining at Animal House

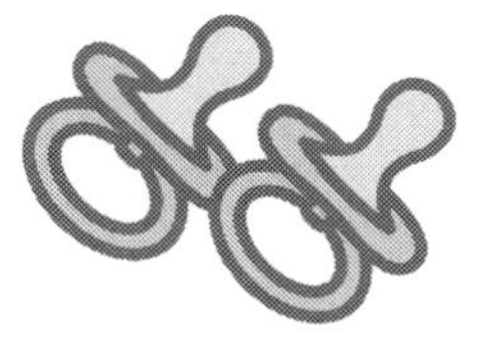

Once your babies have moved through the transition to solid foods and are starting to sit up and eat foods that you might even consider eating yourself, your challenge shifts from the actual feeding to the relentless preparation of their meals. In particular, making dinner every night can become a chore. Sometimes even now, as I stand stymied in front of the open pantry at 5:45 p.m., clueless and sighing, I torture myself by calculating exactly how many dinners I still have to make before the day when they are all eating college cafeteria food and I can pour us two bowls of cereal and call it a night. But what makes this age even trickier for you at dinner time is that your babies are reliably crabby during this "witching hour" and probably won't be understanding about your need to chop and dice vegetables rather than pick them up. The hours from 4–7 p.m. can be a really wild ride, but as with all things twin, the keys are anticipation and preparation.

I don't know any moms of twins who don't own a slow cooker. I'm guessing that about half the stews and casseroles made tonight in this country will be made by mothers of multiples. Slow cookers are perfectly suited to preparing dinner during the babies' afternoon nap and then not thinking about it until it's time to eat. But even the use of slow cookers requires some advance planning, lest you find yourself limited to throwing in whatever you have at hand, possibly resulting in a caper-popcorn-avocado-fish stick ragout. If you aren't the sort of person who plans meals days in advance, it's time to become one.

The meals themselves, however, needn't be elaborate. Convenience still works. There's no rule, for example, that a baby's meal must be cooked, as long as it's edible and nutritious. My babies had plenty of dinners consisting of cottage cheese, apples, hard-boiled eggs, and diced red peppers. And little ones are much more tolerant of leftovers than big ones are; for a while, I tended to cook for the older crowd's later meal and then used the leftovers for the next day's baby meal. Precut vegetables and take-home meals from the grocery store make more sense in your life at this time than they might ever again. So does cooking entrées on Sunday and freezing them for the week.

## Occupying the Kids While You Cook

Eventually I learned that meal preparation was the best time to allow any TV time that would happen that day. I didn't let them watch any TV until they were nearly a year old, and I know that experts would like me to have waited until they were at least two, but those experts never had to get dinner on the table at my house. The twenty or thirty minutes that I let them watch *Sesame Street* videos made our evening meal possible. To this day, that time slot remains our kids' "screen time," once the big girl's homework is finished. Any brain damage they have all experienced as a result has been offset by their having gone to bed fed every night.

If you are trying hard to avoid the television solution, you can think about letting your kids have some "corral time" at this hour, or sitting them in high chairs with some of your baby-safe kitchen utensils to occupy them (stacking cups tend to work better than knives or corkscrews, I find). A friend used to give her baby a teething biscuit to occupy him for the entire meal preparation, not unlike how we leave large marrow bones for our dogs to keep their attention from our shoes and trash when we leave the house for more than ten minutes. Some very brave moms I know actually try to let their babies "help" make dinner. Someday, their kids will steal my kids' spots at Ivy

League schools because of all that interactive learning. And *still* I can live with myself, somehow.

The meal itself can be a bit of a spectacle at this age, too. Your babies' skills with utensils are developing but are fledgling; this, combined with their emerging fascination with cause-and-effect relationships, will result in your picking spoons off the floor fifty times per meal. They will probably think this is much more fun than you will. If you dare to turn your back on them, be prepared to get a sippy cup to the back of the head. Babies' throwing arms can be surprisingly accurate. They will also have difficulty holding on to some foods, so lots of it will cover your floor (to pre-empt this problem, you can roll wet, slippery foods in wheat germ to make them easier to grasp).

When you tell them to stop messing around, they will laugh, and you will begin to believe that you are raising ill-behaved hooligans. Just bear in mind that babies need to feel control over what goes in and what comes out of them (we'll return to this theme in Potty Training Two). It's important to let them play around with all these food textures and test how long you'll play fetch with their spoons. When they demonstrate more interest in inserting their meal in each other's ears than in eating it, just remind yourself that all great scientific discovery starts with basic experimentation. Imagine how much more productive Einstein would have been if only he had had a twin!

# 30

# Napping Nightmares (Yours, Not Theirs)

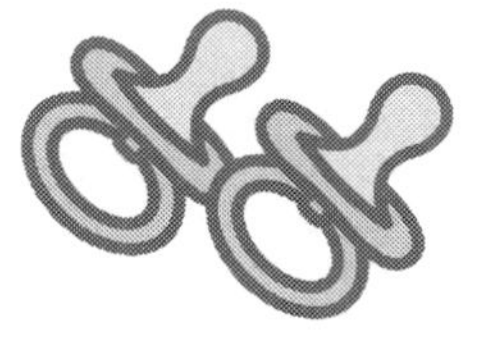

Most twins, including the boy-girl sets, share a bedroom when they are babies, and the vast majority continue to do so well into childhood. There are ample reasons to have twin babies in one room, not the least of which is that their parents may not have had two spare rooms available when they became pregnant with twins. The one major detriment to this arrangement happens right around this age, however. Even though babies this age usually manage to sleep right through any nighttime crying from their siblings, they do tend to be awakened easily during naps. As a result, whenever one baby stirs, the entire naptime is a wash for the whole crew. This scenario will drive you out of your head as you are trying to establish a nap schedule, so it's best to take the preemptive strike of separating them by putting one in another crib, in another room. We did this as long as our boys napped, even when they were old enough to understand their rotation between "crib days" and "Mama's room" days.

Napping in general takes longer to establish than does solid nighttime sleeping, and getting two kids to sleep during the day takes work. Rituals are crucial, just as they were with nighttime sleep training. White noise created by table fans in each room also helped with nap preservation. Good naps are intricately related to good nighttime sleep, which means that crummy naps lead to crummy night sleep, and vice-versa. This illogical truth plays itself out repeatedly: a rested kid falls asleep and stays asleep easily at the next sleep time; an overtired kid tends to have disturbed, messy sleep, if he gets to sleep at all. Thus, getting two kids into a "restful" pattern in which they are both going down easily and staying down until rested becomes the goal, and achieving it takes dedication, forethought, and some luck.

## High Holy Naptime

The dedication part involves the declaration of the High Holy Naptime as sacred, protected time that won't be sacrificed under any circumstances. The work boils down to sticking to a napping schedule for the weeks or months when your kids are resisting going down or are waking after 45 minutes though you know they need more sleep. The luck part has to do with their falling in synch with the same pattern of successful naps so that they are not waking each other up and are simultaneously asleep long enough for you to have a few precious minutes to yourself. Stick with following your established sleepy-time rituals, and get them down in their cribs at the standard naptimes of 9 a.m. and 1 p.m.—preferably without nursing first. Eventually, your dedication will pay off, and many months of reliable napping will follow. That is one fat payoff for your efforts, so keep at it.

A year or so from now, though, naps will again get tricky. First of all, you will at some point have to let your little animals out of their crib cages and put them in big-kid beds. This will give them license to roam the room, if not the house, when they are supposed to be sleeping. Most kids won't take off at night (though I have known some who will, so be sure to lock the front door when you go to bed), but many toddlers see naptime as optional once they are out of their cribs and in their own beds. Mine used to pad silently from their beds to where I was working and stand there stone silent until, vaguely and suddenly perceiving a small figure near me, I would scream before I could stop myself. That was fun. It will become clear to you that some of their new "inability to nap" during that stage

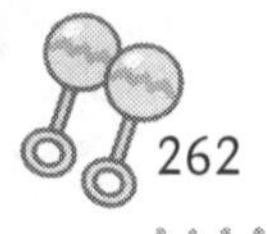



is something more like a disinterest in behaving for *you* when your little demons fall to sleep immediately at their first preschool nap, lying on a hard mat with no blackout shades in the room and ten other preschoolers keeping them company. It will hurt when you ask the teacher what her secret is and she tells you that she told them to go to sleep, so they did. Try not to take it too hard.

Before that happens, you should be granted many months of at least one, and, for a while, two good naps from them every day. For their sake and yours, don't give up on establishing these naps, though the process can take a long time and can be extraordinarily frustrating. They need the sleep, and you need the breaks. Stick with it.

# 31

# Talk, Talk, Talk: Language Acquisition and Twins

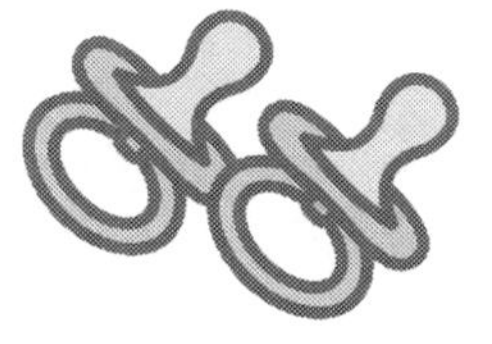

Twins are known to develop language skills more slowly than singletons, generally. Many researchers have suggested probable causes of twin speech delay: twins' tendency to operate in a small world of talk, occupied only by themselves and a caregiver; the likelihood of their socializing less than singletons might with children outside of the home; our own tendency to address twins as one, rather than speaking to them individually; and the development of "twinspeak" between them, making it less necessary for them to attempt new words or sentence structures. Interestingly, research shows that this delay in language development is *not* related to obstetric issues associated with delivering twins.

> If your twins are identical, they are likely to share the same trajectory of verbal development, and if they are fraternal (sharing 50 percent of their genetic makeup, just as any siblings do), their development may vary a bit more.[1]

Keep in mind that a delay in learning language does not necessarily indicate difficulty with reading later or with any other learning issues, for that matter. However, if you anticipate that your twins may learn to speak more gradually than your other children

---

1. University Of Washington, "Twin Study—Genetics Key Factor In Speech Learning," *ScienceDaily* (October 23, 1998), http://www.sciencedaily.com/releases/1998/10/981023073445.htm (accessed December 14, 2007).

did or their peers will, you can adopt practices that will encourage them to develop their language skills to their full capability.

- Be certain that each child has time alone with you every day and that during that time, you are either reading or talking to him or her. The rest of the time, when you are all together, be certain that you have each child's attention when you speak to him or her. Make and try to retain eye contact, address each child by name frequently, put your face close to the child's face when you are talking, ask lots of questions, and wait for answers.
- Work deliberately on word acquisition by repeating what your baby says clearly and slowly and then adding to it. If he asks, "Go store?" answer, "Yes, we are going to the store," rather than, "Yes, we will." Reiterate their words in order to confirm and consolidate them in their minds.
- Try not to slip into a distracted silence when you are home alone with the babies. Though they can entertain each other, they cannot teach each other to speak. Most of their language is going to come from you. So talk a lot. Talk to them, and talk out loud to yourself.
- Be the play-by-play color commentator to your own day. "And now Mama is going to take the cheese out of the refrigerator so that we can make lunch. And look! There's the Chardonnay! But Mama needs to wait a few hours for that, doesn't she? Can you say *Chardonnay?*"

# 32

# Life in the Fat Lane Redux: Time to Get Off the Couch

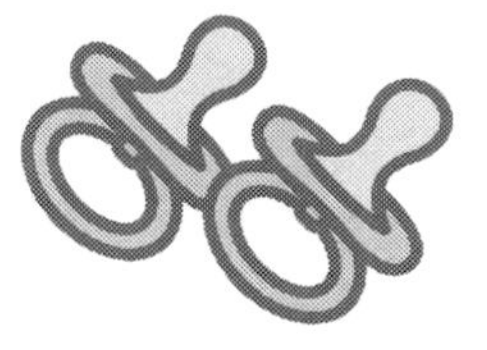

It's time. Your grace period is officially ending. At some point in the second half of your twins' first year, your body will have done just about all it can do on its own to get you back to your former shape. The rest is up to you. Once your weight has hit a plateau below which it will not descend, you've got to get serious about stepping up the exercise program and watching what you eat a bit more carefully. Before you get dismayed, however, think about how great you are going to feel when you're back in shape. If you weren't in good shape in the first place, now is the time to pay a little attention to yourself. The fitter you become, the more you will be able to model a healthy lifestyle for your children, keep up with them, and cope with the daily stresses of raising children.

I recently spied an Internet message board discussion between mothers of twins concerning whether or not to get tummy tucks. One thing we seem to have in common is that our bellies have all been deemed federal disaster areas. Those who had C-sections seem to have a particularly hard time recognizing their abdomens as their own, particularly when there has been separation of abdominal muscles. Even when we get ourselves back into decent shape, most of us still seem to sport aprons made out of our own skin and navels that resemble, for lack of a better analogy, a cow's anus. Not pretty. Plenty of moms of twins have owned up to answering this midsection catastrophe with a tummy tuck. On the other hand, those of us whose bellies were never exposed to the public in the first place other than in medical settings are saving our money for tropical vacations during which we will wear one-piece swimsuits. My elephant-skin belly is a badge of honor, and as long as all that skin doesn't get filled with too many fat cells, I can live with it.

## It's Simple: Eat Less and Move More

We all know the sad truth that there is no magic here. The only way to lose weight is to eat less and move more. So try the basics before you let yourself get excited about a celebrity personal trainer's book promising ten pounds dropped per week if you eat only fruits beginning with the letter *P* on Mondays, followed by only processed meat products on Tuesday, and so on. Carefully plan what you will eat every day. Stick with the plan. Write it down. Simple. It's the same with the exercise: have a plan and stick with it. Put your head down and do it. Don't obsess and don't let yourself say you'll start tomorrow, or after the weekend, or after the staff party, or when the weather is nice.

> Look, what you have been doing for more than a year—carrying and then raising twins—is *so much harder* than sticking to a diet and exercise regimen. This is something you can do. So do it.

It's always better to buddy up with someone else trying to get in shape, so find a partner who will expect you at the gym or at the corner for a run at a particular time. If it is tough for you to limit your calories or if you need some counseling on how to eat well, nothing beats Weight Watchers for educating, inspiring, and guiding you to a healthy weight. Find a local meeting. Once you are committed, you then need to get your partner on board with coverage of the kids—as in every day—in order for you to exercise and meet this goal. Demand it. That's not just fair...it's the least you can ask for the hard labor you've put in. Moreover, it will have benefits for the entire family as you become healthier and more energetic.

Be prepared for a bit of a slog at the beginning. You may be in the worst shape of your life, after all. You've simply got to make a promise to yourself and wake up each day with the same goal, as fresh and compelling and immediate to you as it was the moment you decided you were ready to get in shape. Make this goal a nonnegotiable, unchangeable, predetermined fact that simply does not *get* revisited. In other words, don't wake up every morning and reconsider the goal, reshape it, decide to start working on it tomorrow, or worse, pretend it never existed. The idea is to put in the hard work that is required each day to continue to keep this promise.

As long as you get up every morning with a renewed commitment to your goal, there will be improvements, and at some point, the whole thing will take on a life of its own and you will find yourself unable to function well without your exercise. So be patient. Soon enough, the day will come when you go for a run and, with each step, your butt lands at the same time that each foot does, rather than a half-second later.

As you get deeper into the morass of middle age, you may also begin to realize that maintaining a healthy weight and exercising are no longer about vanity. Now it's all about staying healthy and staying alive as long as you can to take care of these children and their children, too. That should be even more compelling than feeling cute again.

# 33

# Raising Two Individuals

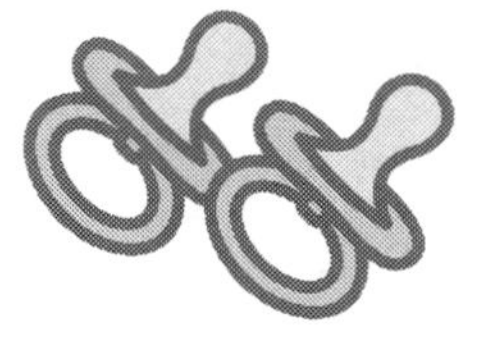

Growing up is a combination of discovering and creating who we are. Identical twins are popular subjects in scientific research because their shared genetics generally mean that any significant differences come from something other than their genetic makeup. They are the perfect nature-nurture laboratory... sort of. It is actually difficult to ascertain the degree to which a child's personality traits are reinforced and perhaps exaggerated by the reactions she gets from others. If, for example, a twin is constantly labeled "the quieter one" for ease of identifying her, who's to say she won't become even more shy as she absorbs that label into her own emerging sense of self?

Although it's easy to advise against comparing twins, it's nearly impossible to do this in reality. We humans tend to make meaning through comparisons. In order to persuade someone of your points in an argument, you instinctively give comparative examples. We name things in relation to each other in order to give them scale, degree, and identity. Meaning is made through named relation—through comparison. If it is our tendency to do this with unrelated concepts, then of course we do it with the most closely related, and twins are arguably more closely related than anything in the world. It will be challenging for you to avoid comparing them, and most of your family and friends won't even bother trying not to do so. "Who's the more athletic one?" they will ask. "She is more outgoing than he is, right?" "Who came out first?" "Who talks more?" These questions may seem insensitive to your children, but they are natural to ask

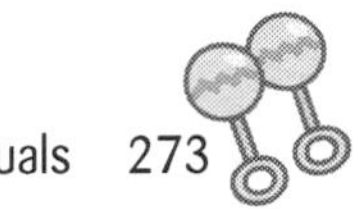

and generally come from a kind and genuine curiosity. In fact, they can be seen as attempts to see the *differences* between your children in order to know each of them as an individual. Often, "comparing twins" is in fact an attempt to *contrast* them.

It is of course important to the development and mental health of each child that you work to encourage his or her uniqueness. You can do this by remembering to separate the kids whenever possible, for example:

- Take one on an errand while the other stays home.
- Consider splitting them into different classrooms in school (many states do this as policy).
- Be sure never to give collective prizes or collective punishments.
- Buy them completely different toys, rather than two of the same in different colors.
- Address them by name whenever you talk to them.
- Enroll them in preschool so that they socialize with other kids.
- Dress them entirely differently.
- Give them separate bedrooms, separate playdates, individual baby scrapbooks, and their own turn to select a favorite dinner or bedtime story.
- Give them each a cake on their birthday, and you may even want to celebrate on different days, with two different parties.

But in the end, you can't entirely take the twin out of twinship, and this is good. Your twins were born married. Perhaps just like you, they will sometimes experience momentary flashes of wishing they weren't married. But overall, they will probably be as happy not to be single as you are. (Aren't you? If not, skip ahead to "Twins and the Potentially Single Mother.")

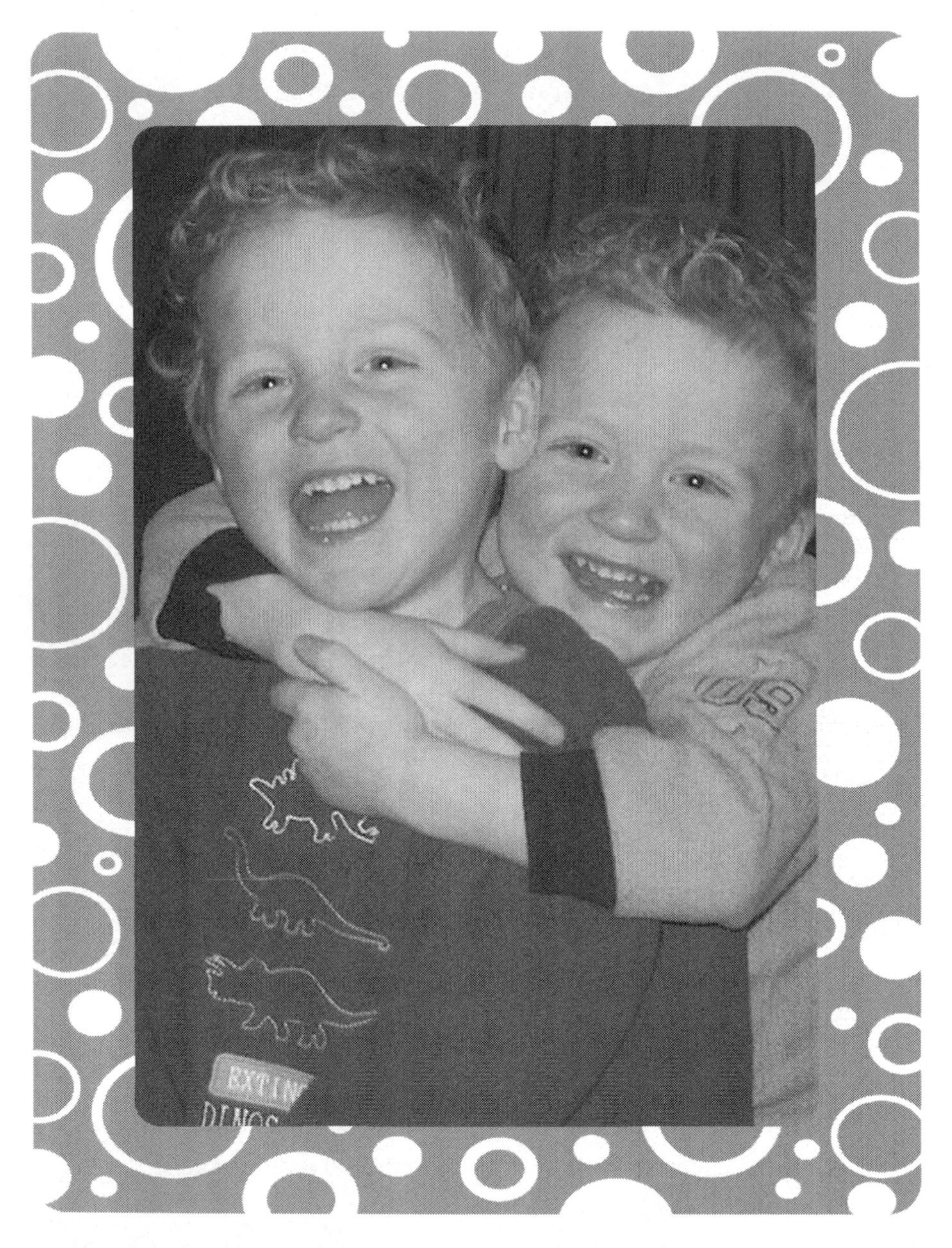

Most older twins say the occasional disadvantages of being a twin are outweighed by the joy of having a soul-mate.

Photo courtesy of the Regan-Loomis family

# Part VI
# Toddlers and Beyond: Herd Mentality

You've done it! You have graduated! Your babies are little people now. They can walk to the car and pull on a shirt and help build a snowman and go to birthday parties. The stroller now spends more time in the garage than the car. Seemingly suddenly, your "babies" are able to pee in the potty, finish a puzzle, use a napkin, and make mini-municipalities with Legos. As you travel out in the world together, you look more like a family and less like a gypsy caravan every day.

My friends with college-age kids tell me that every stage their children have moved through has shed some of the challenges of the last but brought new and unimagined ones to replace them. It's just nature's way of making sure we don't get too good at any one element of parenting; just as we have a challenge in hand, it disappears. The toddler stage certainly presents fresh ways to exasperate and exhaust you, but its highlights outshine its lowlights by far. It's a "good trade" stage. Yes, you'll have to deal with potty training, but guess what? That's right! They can then go to the bathroom to pee! Yes, they throw fits, but most of them are hilarious, if you can ignore the volume. Yes, territorial skirmishes are more common between twins at this stage, but you may also get moments such as I had recently, when my twins sat holding hands next to each other in their car seats and one of them told the other, "You is my best friend." Daily moments like this with your twin toddlers will make you realize that it has all been worth it.

# 34

# Getting Out as a Herd

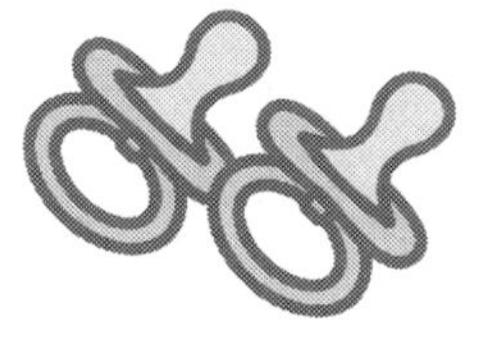

Once your kids are walking and the family is beginning to step back into circulation in the wider world, some of the tradeoffs happen. The pile of baby gear that you need to schlep through the airport will shrink, for example, but so will your kids' ability to hang out in a stroller peaceably while you wait to board a plane. There's a long, wearying stretch of months when your babies are too big to be carried in infant car seats but still too young to walk with you out to the car. Meanwhile, they are growing heavier and harder to carry. The first time that you are able to carry one while the other waddles her own little way to the car, holding on to your free hand, will be a hallelujah moment. From there, it is only a matter of months until you can step from the house, say, "Everyone in the car, please!" and stand there astonished as they clamber into their car seats and start buckling themselves up.

In order to get twins and a sibling or two out of the house in the morning, you can employ a few logistical tricks to make the process one that doesn't leave you panting and in a full sweat by the time you start the car. Once again, you need a plan.

- Before you even set the alarm clock the night before, have a schedule in mind with times that everyone needs to be awake and job assignments for all adults and big kids. Include everything from when everyone needs to be dressed to who will feed the dog.
- Pack lunches and snacks the night before and pop them in the refrigerator.

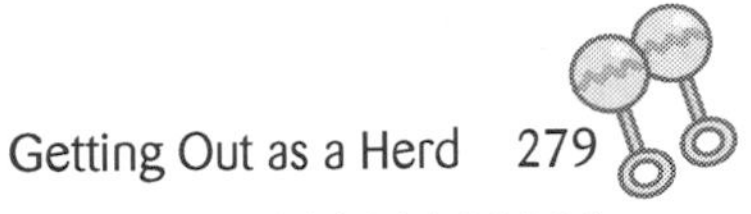



- Lay out everyone's clothes. Hanging clothes organizers with slots for outfits for each day of the week can be a godsend, particularly once kids get to the age of arguments over outfit choices; this way, all those negotiations can be settled on Sunday.
- Have each child's bag—be it a school backpack or a diaper bag—packed and ready to go before bed.
- Put the bags next to the door, along with each child's shoes. One tiny missing shoe five minutes before departure will absolutely sabotage an otherwise seamless exit operation.

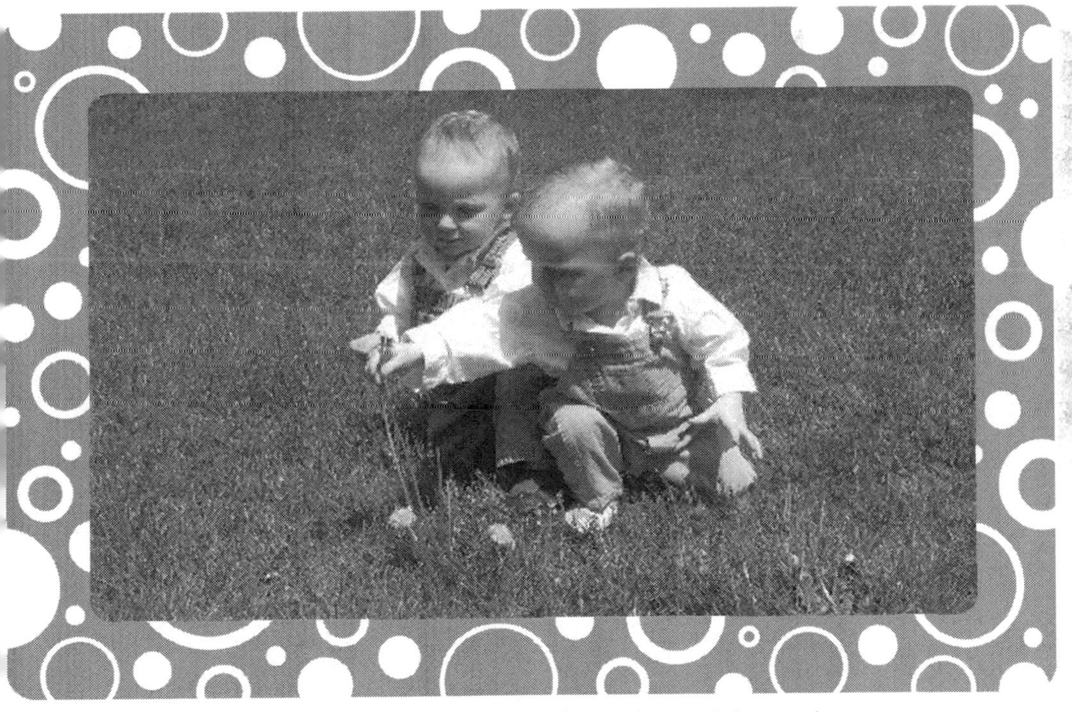

Once they are on the move, twins often explore and play together, moving in tandem like birds, wing to wing.

Photo courtesy of the Regan-Loomis family

In the morning, adults should get up and shower twenty minutes before the kids typically wake up, so that both are ready to deal with the children when they arise. Kids should bathe the night before.

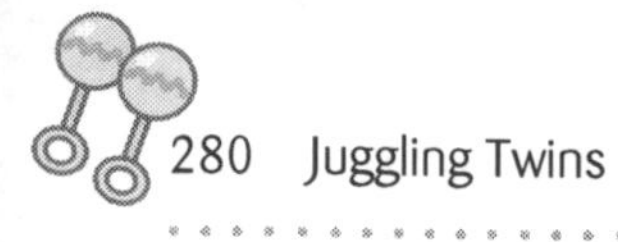


Weekday breakfasts don't need to involve cooking. These can be toast and cereal days, and the homemade waffles and eggs can wait until Saturday. Each day, have a contest to determine which kid has been most helpful. The winner gets a sticker; three stickers get a prize. While you may not want to go so far as to make the kids sleep in their school clothes (don't laugh—I know of a family that does), anything you can do to cut a few minutes here or there will lessen the chances of your having an episode of screaming before the clock strikes 7 a.m.

We stopped brushing our kids' hair years ago and see no reason to start again before they are driving themselves to school. Other families with twins make breakfast a vehicular dining experience, tossing cereal bars and dry toaster waffles back to the kids on the way to drop-offs. Whatever your rules, the more established the routine becomes, the more cooperation you're going to get. Incentives always help. Your kids will stare blankly or perhaps burst into tears when you yell, *"Get in the stupid car right now or you're going to make me lose my job and we'll be living on the streets by next week!"* but just watch how a simple, calm, "First one in the car gets licorice" will rocket them into position.

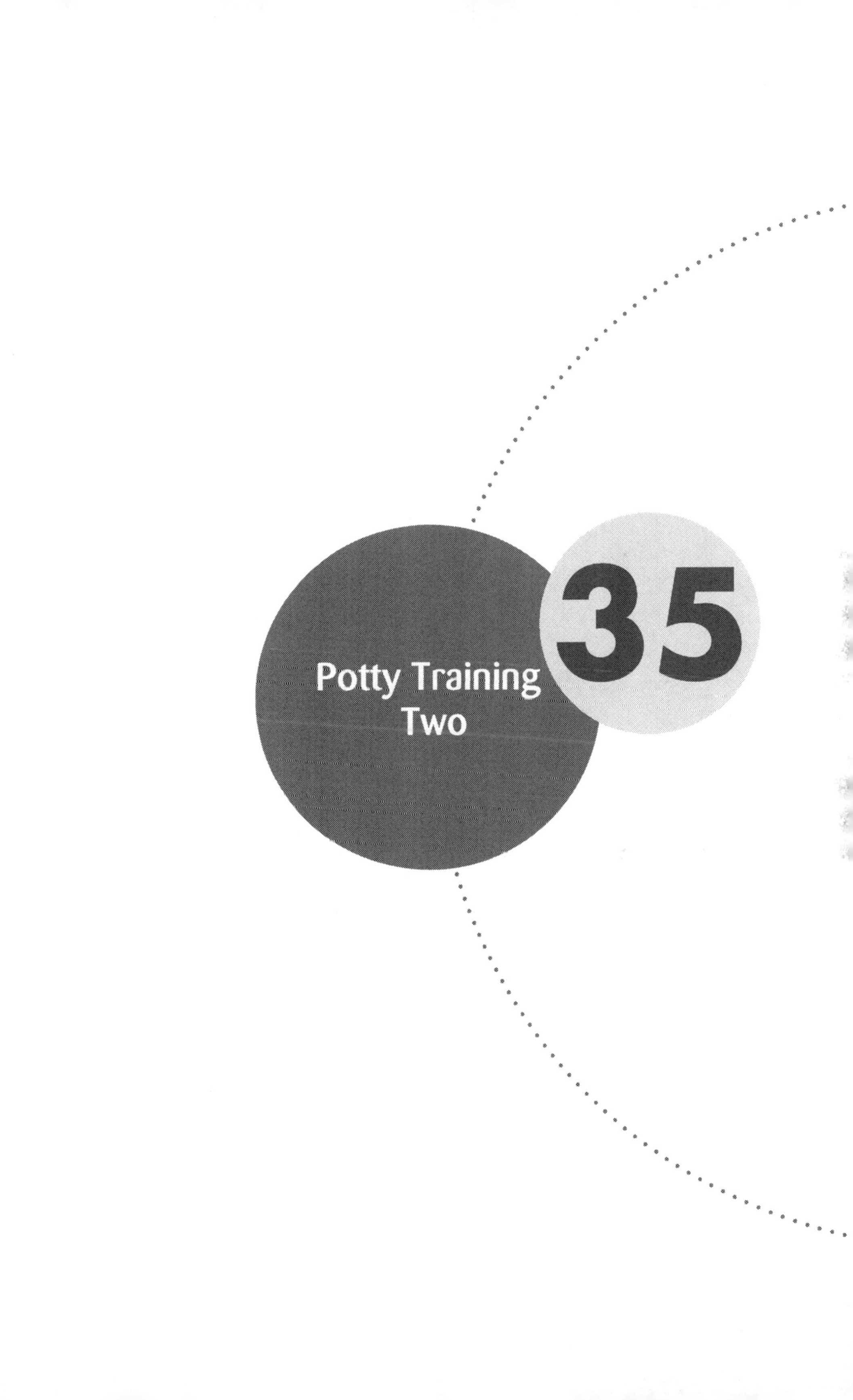
35
Potty Training
Two

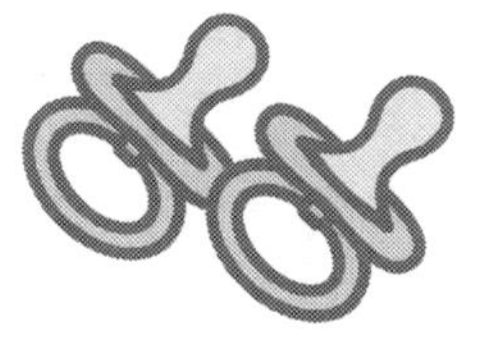

Some aspects of raising twins aren't much different from raising singletons. Here's one: potty training is a disgusting, tiresome, nasty business. There's just no getting around that fact. Gross with one, gross with two. I salute all of you moms who claim to have done it overnight ("We just ran out of diapers, and I told them from now on it was time to use the potty, and they never had an accident!") or whose kids simply decided it was time ("They woke up dry one morning and that was that!"). With buttoned lip, I resist my urge to say to you, "Shut *up,*" though truly, I just can't even construe those scenarios as remotely true. For us, it has been a brutal business both times around. Don't lose faith, though. I have plenty of advice on this topic. I simply can't follow any of it.

I have been a direct eyewitness to the truth of the formula that the less you pressure a child, the more likely it is he will master this and do it in the way you're tempted to pressure him to do it—in the toilet, and with a little warning. Nonetheless, I have been a lousy practitioner of this simple truth. Hopefully, you will be better at this than Yours Truly, who just can't keep quiet when a child does the "I Haffa Go" Dance around the house with no apparent flight plan toward the bathroom. With one of my boys, I harped for a full week, "Really, honey, you need to get in there...I can see you need to go... how about if I help you?" only to have the child stop and stare right at me as he pooped his pants.

"It okay now, Mama. I not haffa go anymore," he would tell me, ever so sweetly.

Finally, somehow, I took the leap of faith and let him figure it out on his own.

And guess what? Just like the experts say, the minute I said, "Do whatever you need to do," both kids marched to the bathroom and took care of business. Learn from my mistakes before you, too, spend a week at home doing soiled little-people laundry, petrified to take your children out in public.

Though I did a stellar job of making it unnecessarily difficult both times through this process, I have to say it was in fact easier the second time around, with twins. This is not because I had experience the second time through—I did it pretty much all wrong both times. It was easier with our twins simply because we did at least have the small blessing of peer pressure working its magnetic magic. Just as kids in preschool watch slightly older kids toddling off to the potty all day and start to get the idea a bit earlier than those at home might, so too, when one twin gets it, the second one may fall in step. Ours essentially learned the same day.

Peer pressure can work in reverse, however, and one twin may resist *because* the other has done it. Don't assume that just because one of your twins is ready, the other must also be. A leading urologist told us that the singular point to remember about potty training is to *let the child make the call* on when he or she is ready. It follows that each individual child must do this for him- or herself, and that one twin's readiness should not force the other's hand. Your twins may figure this out on the same day, as mine did, or they may do so a full year apart.[1] As they say, neither is right or wrong—just differently ready for the transition.

1. Anecdotal observation suggests that same-sex twins are probably more likely to be simultaneously ready to learn than are fraternal, and that identicals are most likely.

## Reality Check

Perhaps my view of potty training is tainted by the fact that we had a 90-pound, ill-behaved puppy in the family during the potty-training period and my role as the Remover of Others' Accidents was simply getting to me. In the end, I will also recall that period somewhat more fondly as being filled with days of hustled rock-hopping from public toilet to public toilet, asking the kids at every turn if they needed "to go." Fortunately, I had already memorized the location of every public toilet in town during my pregnancy, so we were never far from relief.

# 36

# Twins and the Single Mother

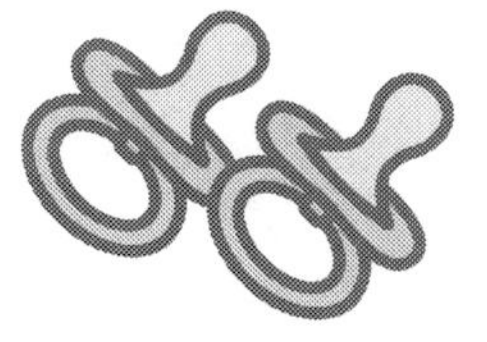

Just as strung-out, overwhelmed parents of single babies can't imagine what it would be like to have twins, married parents of twins can't imagine what it would be like to try to raise twins alone. The mandates to ask for and accept help, to swallow pride, and to reach out are even more crucial for a mom trying to do this on her own than for one with a co-parent on the scene.

If you were never married, you have at least been spared the additional stress of an ongoing divorce and the complex emotions unleashed by that process (or the anguish of having been widowed with young children). You also have the benefit of being able to make all the calls regarding the upbringing of your kids. If you don't want your kids learning to hunt, they won't. No discussion; no negotiation. At the same time, you also don't get any significant breaks from child care. A divorced or divorcing mom with shared custody at least has the probability of a brief respite at regular intervals.

One divorced friend of ours claims that the end of her marriage afforded her some surprising and unusual time for herself, since her ex-husband had never taken responsibility for the kids when they were together. Now, she had every other weekend to herself, which she hadn't experienced since she was twenty years old and single. That's a slightly tarnished silver lining to a situation that doesn't offer many other obvious advantages.

Raising children alone is a difficult proposition no matter what; raising twins alone is tough not just because of all the usual challenges associated with single parenting—exhaustion, loneliness, and financial strain, for starters—but also for logistical reasons. If one child is sick, both are going with you to the pediatrician. If you need to take the trash to the dump, the kids are coming, too. If the car needs to be repaired, you'll need a loaner; if you have more than the two children, you may need a loaner that fits three car seats in the back. If you're flying with the children, you are juggling the luggage and kids by yourself. Any time you are driving with them, everyone must get out to go to the bathroom at a rest stop, even if only one of you has to go. Seven-year-old boys come with you into the women's restroom. Simple outings become inordinately complicated.

The edict that "you can't do this alone" is true for single moms, too, though they are in a sense doing that every day. If you are to remain healthy enough and happy enough to provide constant care for your twins, you have to be able to find help in order to rejuvenate somehow. Join Mothers of Twins. Call on friends. Join a temple or a church. (If you're agnostic or atheist, find a Unitarian Universalist church—they can work with that!) Your situation may warrant more concern than that of a single mother of two or more kids of different ages, though that is in itself an extremely demanding circumstance. People will want to help, if you are able to get yourself to reach out. They don't necessarily have to come and take over all your Saturday duties. Just sitting in the house with sleeping babies on a weeknight will allow you a chance to get out of the house alone.

If you can afford it, you should feel justified in using every possible purchasable convenience or service, from grocery and dry-cleaning delivery to regular babysitting hours during which you can exercise. Most states also have programs designed to help foster the health and education of children; don't hesitate to contact social work agencies if you are struggling. Understandably, an acquaintance who raised her twins alone reports that "there is nothing I am more proud of than raising my girls alone. It's the hardest and the best thing I've ever done."

## Twins and the Potentially Single Mother

Everybody knows that marriage is hard work. Holding a marriage to its dreamy wedding-day promises takes an array of skills that many people haven't yet perfected. That's before you add kids, that's before you add the stress of having two children at once, and that's before you *take away* shared free time or the energy to reconnect.[1] After all those calculations, one can see why the basics of marital maintenance are more dramatically necessary for a couple with twins than for "normal" married people. It's small wonder that divorce is a sadly common topic of discussion at Mothers of Twins meetings.

Like working out or taking care of yourself, marriage can appear to be one of those elements of your life that can wait for attention until the twins are a bit more in hand. You tell yourself—or perhaps you even tell your partner—that when the crisis period is over, then we can really "focus on us again." But attempting to compartmentalize your life like this can't work, really, because the crisis of these babies needs your marriage to be in good shape now. The babies need you to work as a team just as much as you do, and they can't wait, even if you think *you* can. Putting a relationship on hold while you concentrate on the babies is impossible. Marriage is not static; if you are not nurturing the relationship, it is degenerating.

---

1. While marriage longevity may benefit from a couple's desire to stay together "because of the kids," the stresses associated with child-rearing have also been linked with decreased satisfaction in marriage over time, most recently in correlation with the onset of puberty for first and second children. Depressing, huh? See Shawn D. Whiteman, Susan M. McHale, and Ann C. Crouter, "Longitudinal Changes in Marital Relationships: The Role of Offspring's Pubertal Development," *Journal of Marriage and Family* 69, no. 4 (2007): 1005–20, doi:10.1111/j.1741-3737.2007.00427.x.

Most parenting experts tell you to make time for yourselves, to foster your relationship with date nights and rekindle the romance with back rubs. That's great, but if you're not speaking to each other by the time date night arrives, either because you're so pissed off or because you have become so disconnected that you can't think of anything to talk about, then even a shared flambé dish won't do much rekindling. Beyond relationship remediation through dates and appointments for sex, think on a daily basis of your marriage and what it needs, and of your spouse and what he or she needs. Yes, this is asking a lot of someone whose plate is crammed full. Yes, taking care of one more person would seem to be just the ticket for putting you over the edge. But the work that goes into fostering a happy marriage pays with interest. If you are functioning as a team, everything else becomes more manageable; if you are instead preoccupied by yet another argument, everything you do today will be more labored. If you are unhappy, everything is simply harder. Besides, you promised you would tend to this marriage and make it last. Remember the "for better, for worse" part? Twins provide plenty of both.

## Traps to Avoid

There are some very predictable traps into which a couple can stumble, hand in hand, when raising twins together. One is the division of labor. Having declared you Boss of the World a while back, I now need to retreat a bit and suggest that you also need to at least *appear* to favor consensus and negotiation. In an ideal world, if you are staying home with the children, you could think of your "day job" as having whatever hours your spouse is away at a real-world day job, and then both of you would share the work of the remaining hours at home.

Because your day job happens to be at the same worksite as this shared portion, however, it might sometimes seem that you are in fact responsible for double shifts every day. That's not fair. It is

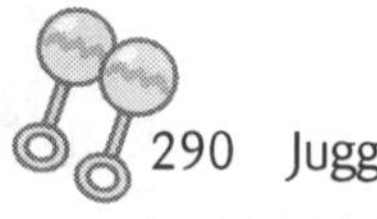


also not fair, however, to expect your partner to understand this rationale if you haven't discussed it. Nor is it fair for you to expect an immediate transition from the outer world to yours as soon as your honey walks through the doorway.

No team works well without great communication. Don't rely on telepathy to make your points. As one friend says, "If I don't tell my husband why I'm upset, he just chalks it up to hormones and waits for it to pass. It never occurs to him that he's the problem."

Another trap that parents of twins are particularly prone to, given the intensity of their families' needs, is the Comparative Workload Trap. We are all big babies sometimes, needing a ton of credit for our hard work and a ton of support when we are struggling. In all likelihood, you are both working extremely hard. It is fruitless to play the "I'm doing more than you are" game when you need that credit or support. First of all, it won't create credit or support; at best, it will produce defensiveness. Secondly, this is not a competition. If you need credit, ask for it. If you need support, ask for it. Directness is more effective than games are, and relative misery is never a useful measure.

A working team acknowledges that each player is participating, each is working hard, and each is deserving of credit. By all means, you should share your daily frustrations with your partner—the one person capable of truly getting it—but do so to vent, not to accuse. And if the workload truly isn't divided fairly, you'll get closer to getting what you need with calm, reasoned discussion than you will with bitter accusations that back your partner into a corner.

If this advice sounds simplistic for situations that are by their nature quite complex, that's because of tennis. When I am playing tennis, a complex game if played well, occasionally some element of my game is off and, as a result, my whole match threatens to unravel. At that point, an experienced player abandons complex strategy and goes back to the basics of bending her knees and watching the ball closely on every shot. When marriages start to unravel, they too can benefit from the practice of returning to the basics—in this case, the basics of being nice to each another—and imagining what the other needs in order to feel cherished. From there, the complexities can be picked at one by one. But the basics come first.

In difficult moments in your marriage, it's too easy to fantasize that there's someone else out there who is perfect and that if only you were out of this relationship, you could find that person who would understand you and know how to pitch in more with these children. But as my friend Carolyn says, "Why would I ever leave my husband? Nobody's perfect, and I would only be trading him in for a new model with his own issues that I'd have to figure out and deal with." I count my lucky stars every day that I married someone who appears to share this sentiment.

# 37

# Having More (No, Seriously!)

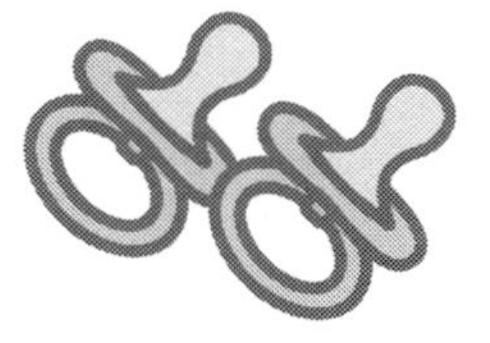

Admit it. Don't you sort of want to have another baby just so you can see how easy it would be to have just one at a time?

Tread carefully! By some estimates, if you have had fraternal twins, you are five times more likely to have another set than is a mom of single babies.[1] If you were to use fertility treatments to help conceive the next child, your relative chances would be even higher than that.

Deciding whether to continue growing your family is a process of assessing risks and probabilities, and many of the questions you'll need to ask yourselves reflect those unknowns. How long would it take to get pregnant? At what point would the twins be more independent? How would they handle having a sibling? Am I getting too old? If I wait, how greatly would my chances of miscarriage increase? If we stop now, will we regret it in five years? Ten years? Can we afford another? Would another child end my career indefinitely? And perhaps, could I handle the challenges of having fertility treatments again?

I know plenty of parents who knew when they were pregnant with twins that there would be no more kids after that. I also know of parents who, having had twins, essentially declared a "we're in it, let's go for it" policy and had big families of four or more kids, in some cases including more than one set of twins. Obviously, only the two

---

1. Peg Plumbo, "Twins: What Are Your Chances of Having a Second Set?" iVillage.com, http://parenting.ivillage.com/pregnancy/pmultiples/0,,midwife_3pdp,00.html (accessed December 23, 2007).

of you know where you are in that range and how you can answer all those questions. The knotty part is that these are timely questions with answers that shift from month to month as everyone in your family ages and changes. I know of a mom who says that it seemed like a good idea to have another baby when her twins were in their second year and getting manageable, but once the baby was born, the twins were nearly three and suddenly going through a more difficult stage of testing her and throwing tantrums. Complicating the decision-making process further is time pressure, since you obviously can't wait forever as you are weighing your options.

If you come up on the "let's go for it" end of the range, you then need to figure out when. No, I don't mean what night you should try, though finding one when you're both awake and willing could indeed be a challenge. I mean what sort of spread in age you are hoping for between the twins and another child. It's better to think in terms of hopes than plans, as we all know; you have only so much control over this, obviously. Our plan had been a two-year spread between our first child and second child; the reality was a five-year spread between our first child and second *children,* punctuated by a devastating late-term loss—of twins—in between. The "decision" to have more children assumes a certain lack of control over the whole prospect. For many of us, that control is a reasonable price to pay for our dreams.

For some families, the hope is to have kids who are as close in age as possible. This desire comes from several perceived advantages over waiting. The thinking starts with: "A baby would pose no major change in our lifestyle at this point. Once the babies are out of diapers, we won't want to start all over again. We're already swimming; let's do it before we come up for air." If you're truly up for it, there are some distinct advantages to this tactic. It is true, for example, that the closer the children all are in age, the better the chances that they will eventually all play together. It would also

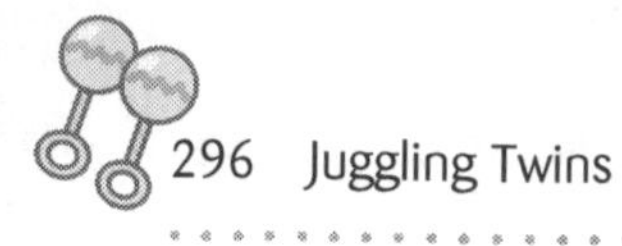


consolidate the demanding first years of child-raising so that they would be finished in a big, blurry blink. The kids would be more likely to attend the same schools at the same time, they would share similar developmental issues (you wouldn't have one signing up for driving lessons while another is potty training), and you would obviously be younger, possibly more energetic parents than you would be if you were to wait.

On the other hand, you might feel calmer and more rested if you waited a while. You might see the prospect of being pregnant while your babies still need to be carried a lot as a nightmare in the making. You could very reasonably wonder if having three in diapers won't be a bit much to handle. Waiting also has some distinct advantages, in spite of its making the conception process trickier as your biological clock winds down. If you have another child when your twins are of an age when they can play independently, hop into their car seats independently, and use the toilet, you may be afforded bonding time with the new baby that you felt deprived of with the twins. And yes, it is inevitable that you will find one baby easier than the twins were.

> As for the closeness of the kids, as a "caboose," born when my siblings were twelve, ten, and eight, I can attest that I am much closer to my siblings than are many of my friends with siblings who are closer to them in age. There is something to be said for not having to compete with siblings. With our kids, the five-year spread has worked out beautifully, and we could not ask for a more wonderful sister than our eldest has become to her beloved brothers.

A year or so after their twins were born, our friends Jason and Wendy decided to have a third baby. Wendy says, "I love that there are just two years between them all. We had always thought we would have three, and we were in the whirl of caring for babies, so we just went for it. You definitely pay a price for a while, but there are immense rewards on the other side. Each of them always has a buddy because they're so close in age. It's nice that we can all do things together and that they like a lot of the same books, same shows, and same activities. There were definitely moments of 'What were we thinking?' But, you know, sometimes it's better not to think so much. Honestly, I don't even know how we did it. I can't remember. But we did it, and I can tell you that I have never once heard my children say, 'I'm bored.' " Neither are Jason and Wendy.

# Conclusion: Pressing the Pause Button

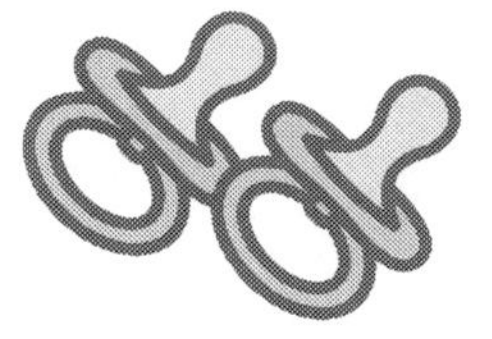

Did this happen to you as it did to us? As we were leaving the hospital with our two beautiful newborn babies, we waited for the elevator with other parents of newborns. Looking around at the other parents, both of us were independently struck by the same emotion: *pity*. What a rip-off for them, we thought. They only got one.

It is difficult to be grateful for water when you are drowning. Similarly, we parents of twins can easily lose sight of the miracle before us when the chaos of our lives is swirling around us. And then, unexpectedly, our attention is jolted back to our blessed status by the vision of our two children hugging each other in the yard, or sleeping side by side with virtually indistinguishable angel faces, or whispering to each other between their cribs. Even when we are used to them, twins unwittingly inspire our awe.

As my peer group has graduated into parenthood, I've noted that there appear to be two camps of thinking about how to integrate children into a couple's life. The first philosophy says that, in essence, the world halts for babies. There will be time later for life as we knew it. Stop and smell the baby heads. The other philosophy says that it's healthier for the kids and us if we retain our lifestyle as best we can, letting them adjust to us. If the couple used to backpack a lot, they get a bigger tent. If they cleaned on Saturdays, kids over two years old get a chore list. Life goes on, but with more participants. Hoping to preserve our lives as we know them, some of us agree to the latter approach when we are contemplating having children, but then can't quite follow through with it once we get a whiff of those baby heads. Our world stops in spite of our plans.

For parents of twins, pausing in order to enjoy their children's early years is both more pressing, because of their miracle status, and more difficult to achieve, because of the bedlam their births have caused. But there are double the moments to observe here: double the love to give and receive, and double the reasons to stop, breathe, and let their perfection wash over you.

Can't the laundry wait?

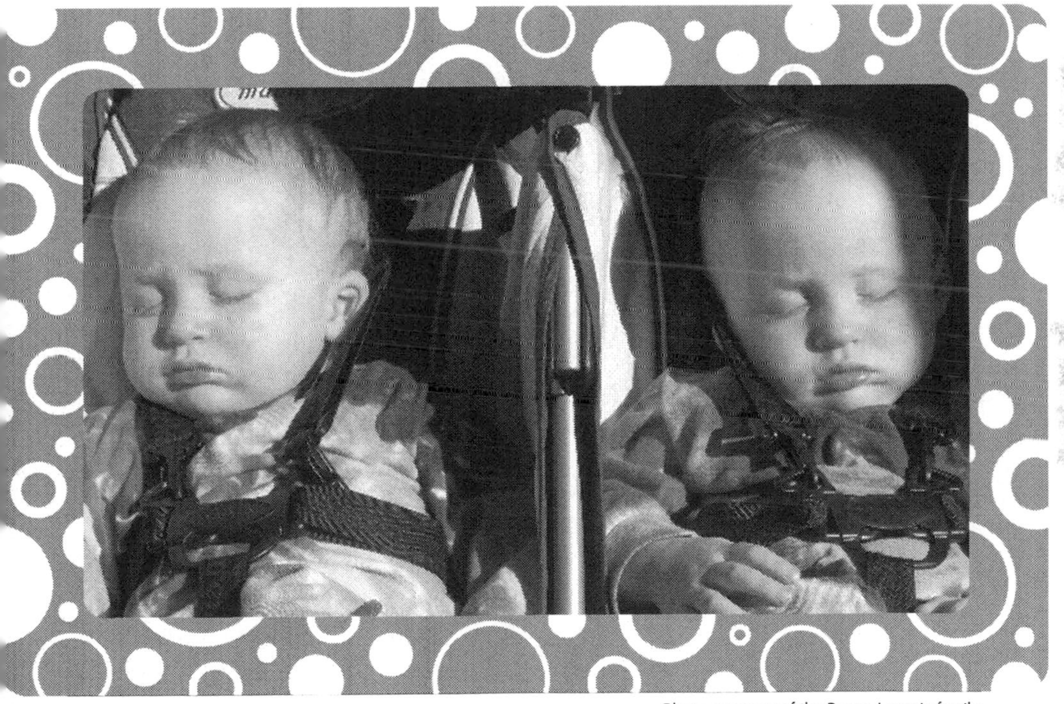

Photo courtesy of the Regan-Loomis family

## Both and Each

The next time we are shopping for tomatoes
And yet another cart-pushing poet succumbs
To the irrepressible need to proclaim "Double Trouble!"
We will try to credit her innate love of rhyme

Rather than a galling lack of judgment
In her getting you so purely wrong.
How could she, after all, envision
The mountain of loss we crawled up and over
On our trek to claim our "trouble"?
How could she know our loss of breath
When you first fastened eyes on one another
And we watched the birth of lifelong love?
How could she imagine the one of you
First smiling at the other, as if in recognition
The world loves twins in the aggregate
But begrudges them their particulars.
It might define you as the "more than he" or "faster than"
Or The One with the Thicker Ear Fold,
But also makes you share the poems it writes you
And fails to call you by your precious names
For fear of rude confusion.
But what offense with coupledom
So perfect as to mingle self and other?
Forgive us, all we single types,
The barbed boundaries we've supposed
Between a *you* and a *me,*
And we will promise you
To love you both and each,
Boy and boy,
Love of our life and love of our life,
The echoing reply
To our redoubled prayers.

—MRL

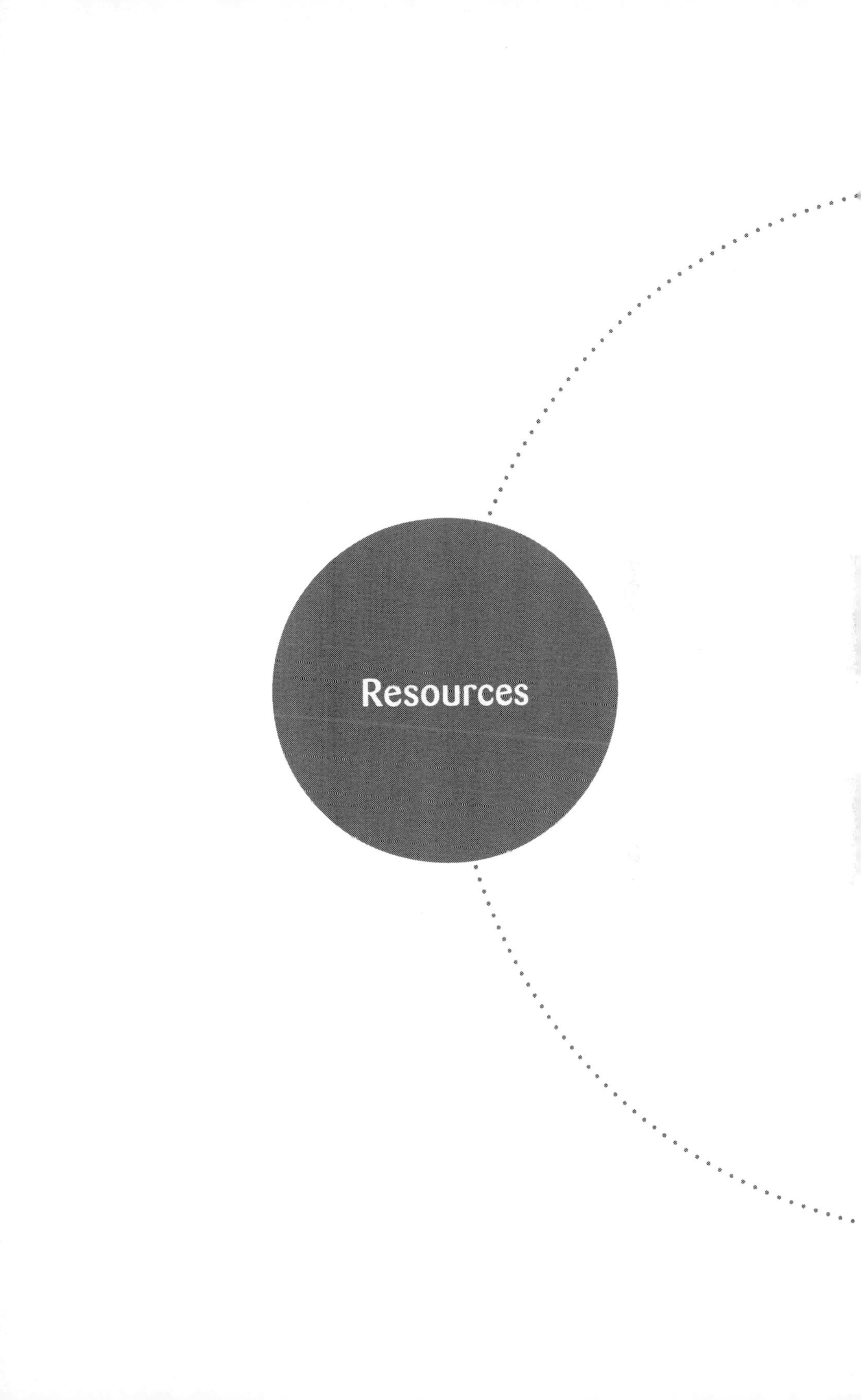

# Resources

## Child Care

http://www.sittercity.com has a huge national database of screened babysitters (and pet sitters, elder care sitters, and house sitters, too) for both long-term and short-term needs. It's a fun site, worth checking out even if you already have help lined up.

http://www.nanny.com, http://www.4nanny.com, and http://www.nannynetwork.com are comprehensive how-to sites on finding and employing a nanny.

## Early Childhood Development

http://www.naeyc.org (National Association for the Education of Young Children) is an organization of early childhood educators promoting improved quality of programs for children from birth to third grade. This website contains a searchable database of NAEYC-accredited programs as well as resources and materials for parents.

http://www.nccic.org/index.html (National Child Care Information Center, sponsored by the U.S. Department of Health and Human Services) has links to child-care resources.

http://www.zerotothree.org (Zero to Three) is a national educational nonprofit organization with links for parents and professionals about child development. Established over thirty years ago, its expertise earned it a federal contract with the Office of Head Start to operate the Early Head Start Resource Center.

## Health

Barbara Luke and Tamara Eberlein, *When You're Expecting Twins, Triplets, or Quads: Proven Guidelines for a Healthy Multiple Pregnancy,* rev. ed. (HarperCollins, 2004). The best book on the topic, hands down.

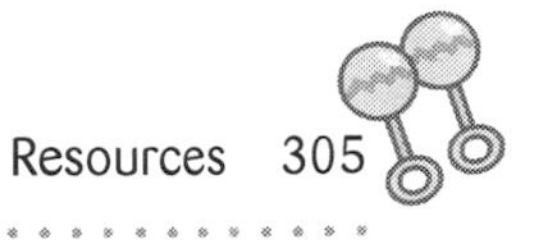

http://www.marchofdimes.com (March of Dimes) provides pregnancy advice and exhaustive information on the prevention of premature birth.

http://www.aap.org (American Academy of Pediatrics) has a "Parenting Corner" with great advice and summaries of current medical recommendations and research.

## Sleep Issues

Marc Weissbluth, *Healthy Sleep Habits, Happy Child* (Random House, 2003).

Richard Ferber, *Solve Your Child's Sleep Problems* (Simon & Schuster, Inc., 1986).

Elizabeth Pantley, *The No-Cry Sleep Solution: Gentle Ways to Help Your Baby Sleep Through the Night* (Contemporary Books, 2002).

## Stuff

http://www.craigslist.com has listings for used equipment in your area. It is also a resource for self-advertising nannies and sitters.

http://www.nurturecenter.com sells "natural parenting products" for babies and moms.

## Support

http://www.nomotc.org (National Organization of Mothers of Twins, Inc.) is the quintessential support group for parents of twins. The site contains links to local chapters to join and meetings to attend.

http://www.mothering.com is the website for *Mothering Magazine*, which advises on "natural family living" and has useful links to research and baby products.

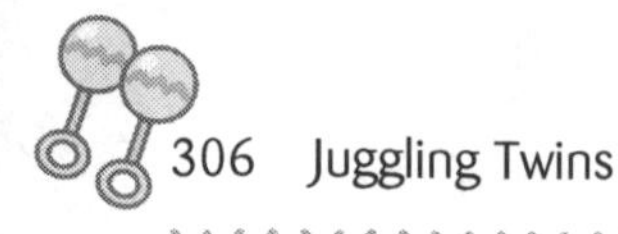


http://www.twinslist.org is a comprehensive site with links to resources and information for all stages of parenting of twin children.

http://www.preemietwins.com is a blog hosting preemie parents' stories and support, and also links to general information about multiples.

## Travel

http://www.jetsetbabies.com and http://www.babiestravellite.com ship supplies to your vacation spot in advance of your arrival so that you don't have to take everything with you.

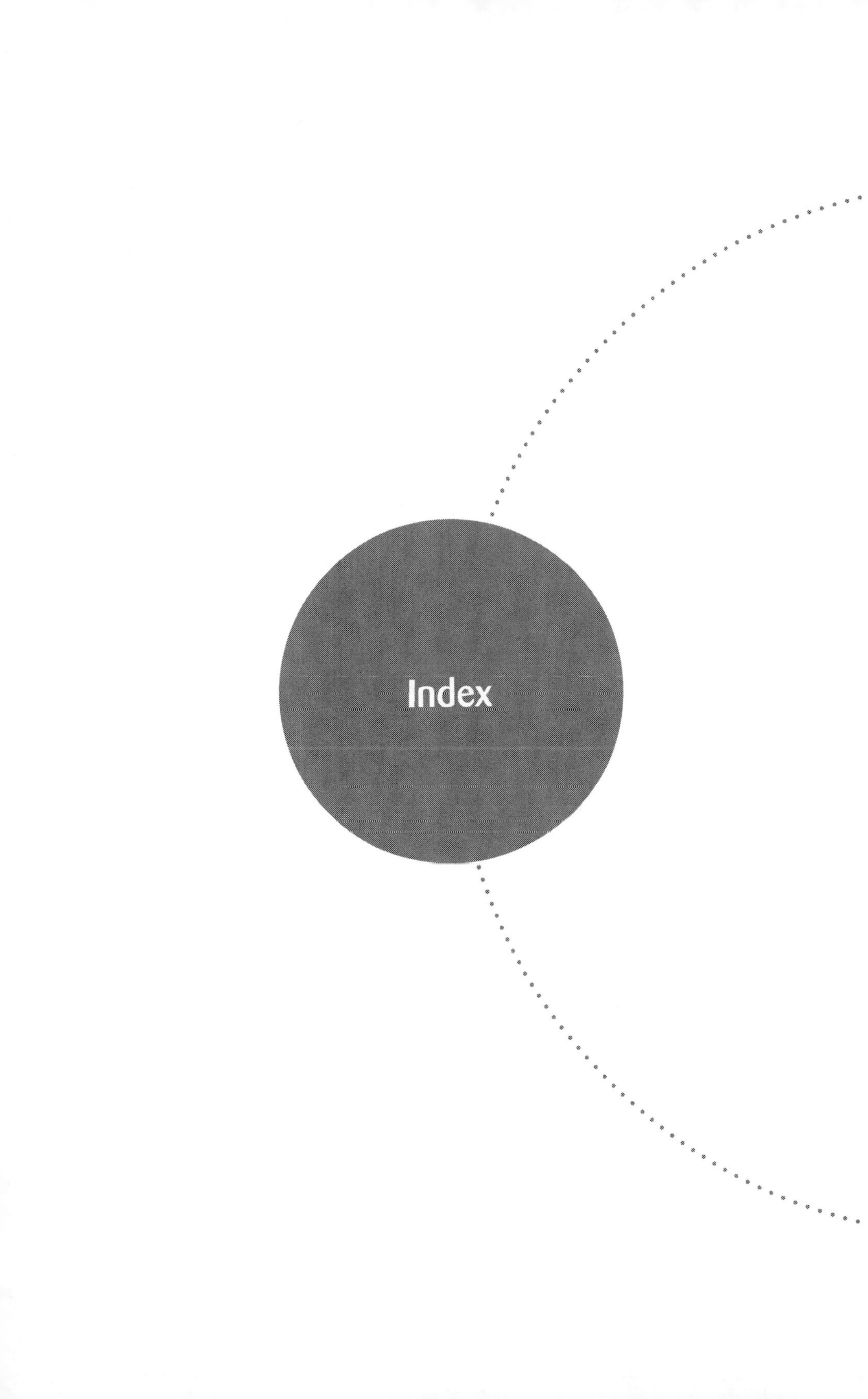

# Index

## A



## B

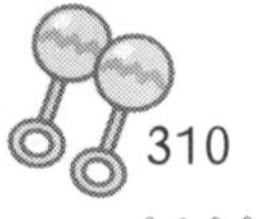




## D



## E

# F

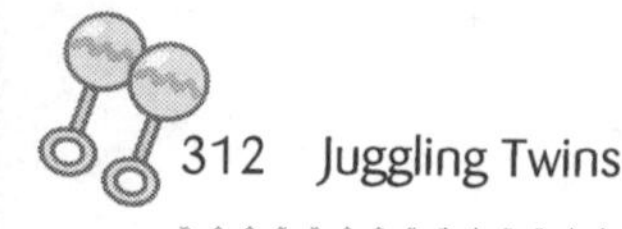




## G

## H



## I



## J

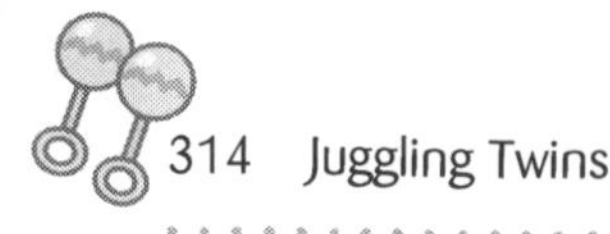


## K



## L



## M

## N

## O



## P

## Q



## R

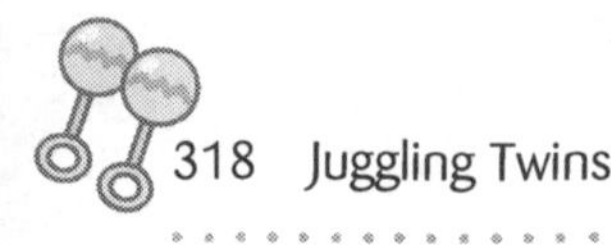

## T

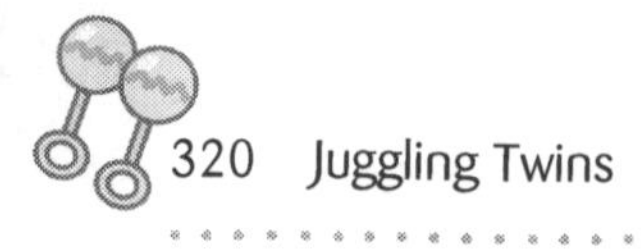




## U



## V

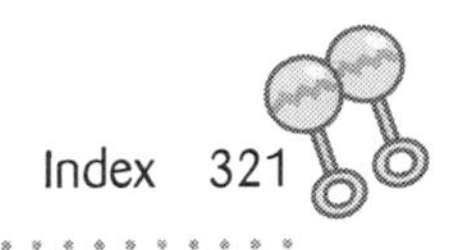

# About the Author

When Meghan Regan-Loomis discovered that she was pregnant with twins, she searched fruitlessly for the book that would explain how to manage the logistics and challenges of caring for two babies at once. Discovering that it didn't yet exist, she vowed that she would figure out the answers and one day write the book herself. A veteran high school English teacher, she specializes in American literature, Shakespeare, Milton, and, more recently, How to Burp Two Babies at Once. A competitive tennis player who received her undergraduate degree from Kenyon College, she lives near Boston with her family.